DR. SONIA'S
GUIDE TO
NAVIGATING
PELVIC PAIN

DR. SONIA'S GUIDE TO NAVIGATING PELVIC PAIN

Result-Oriented Strategies
for Better Quality of Life

Sonia Bahlani, MD

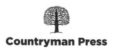

Countryman Press

An Imprint of W. W. Norton & Company
Independent Publishers Since 1923

Dr. Sonia's Guide to Navigating Pelvic Pain is intended as a general information resource for readers. The remedies, approaches, and techniques described in this book are meant to supplement, *not* substitute for, medical diagnosis, care, or treatment and should not be used in lieu of treatment of any diagnosed condition or any symptom that may require the personal attention of a physician. We encourage you to consult a physician or other qualified health care provider before starting a new diet, exercise regimen, or supplement (conventional or otherwise) to determine if it is the right fit for your individual medical needs. Be sure to read the **Foreword** (page ix) for additional important safety guidelines.

Individuals and case examples described in this book are composite portraits representing no particular person, living or dead, and any apparent resemblance of names or descriptions is purely coincidental.

References in this book to third-party organizations, tools, products, and services are also for general informational purposes. Neither the publisher nor the author can guarantee that any particular practice or resource will be useful or appropriate to the reader. The publisher is not responsible for and cannot endorse any website, content, or products other than its own.

For information about permission to reproduce selections from this book, write to Permissions, Countryman Press, 500 Fifth Avenue, New York, NY 10110

For information about special discounts for bulk purchases, please contact W. W. Norton Special Sales at specialsales@wwnorton.com or 800-233-4830

Manufacturing by Lake Book Manufacturing
Book design by Ellen Cipriano
Production manager: Devon Zahn

Countryman Press
www.countrymanpress.com

An imprint of W. W. Norton & Company, Inc.
500 Fifth Avenue, New York, NY 10110
www.wwnorton.com

978-1-68268-686-7 (pbk)

10 9 8 7 6 5 4 3 2 1

For my mother, Pushpa Israni Bahlani, MD
(November 29, 1945–March 12, 2021),
who inspired me to pursue my love for
medicine, who encouraged me to follow my
dreams, no matter where they took me,
and who loved me unconditionally—and
taught me to do the same.

Nothing would be possible
without you.

CONTENTS

CONTENTS

SECTION 3. TREATMENTS

FOREWORD

Clinical medicine is constantly changing. Some therapeutic methods I discuss in this book are off-label strategies, supported by anecdotal data and clinical experiences. And every patient's needs are different.

This book is not meant to represent a comprehensive cohort of clinical care for every chronic pelvic pain patient. It's meant to empower you, the reader, to navigate your own care by helping you understand the known causes and treatment strategies currently available for pelvic pain. I've included a Resources section of sources I've relied on, and which you might find helpful as further reading (see page 202). My ultimate goal is to help those who are suffering find ways to reduce or ideally eliminate their suffering.

If you're dealing with pelvic pain, the first question you probably have is this: How do I feel better? I empathize with your desire to find relief as quickly as possible, but you and your health care providers first need to do your due diligence to uncover the root cause of your pain. My priority in my own practice is to treat the patient, not just their symptoms and this is the approach I advocate in this book. Treatment will help you feel better, but it's only part of a bigger picture. Without first understanding what's causing your symptoms, you can't develop an informed and effective plan. Once your health care provider has investigated your pain and diagnosed your condition and its causes, they can then begin to create a holistic treatment plan, which I firmly believe should incorporate lifestyle consultation, wellness coaching, and actionable strategies and pain management techniques.

If you are reading this book, chances are that your pelvic pain has interfered with your life for long enough. That pain is your body's way of telling you something is wrong. Are you ready to start listening?

INTRODUCTION

When I became a physician, I guess you could say I "went into the family business." I come from a family of physicians, dentists, and pharmacists, so I was immersed in the world of health care from a young age. I grew up watching doctors and nurses go about their day with my mom at the hospital. I spent countless hours with my dad at his office. And I loved it. I knew from early on that I, too, wanted to be a healer. I wanted to take care of people In their darkest moments. I wanted to live a life of purpose and have a direct impact on the lives of others.

And while I've always wanted to be a doctor, I didn't necessarily grow up knowing or understanding the niche of pelvic pain. In fact, my path to where I am today was a long and winding one, with many forks in the road that forced me to choose a direction that would alter my original course. I arrived at one of my biggest turning points in 2012: I had just completed my residency in OB-GYN (obstetrics-gynecology) but felt unsure about my role in clinical medicine. Imagine training your entire life to do something and then thinking, "I'm not sure I want to do this."

I was questioning myself because I hadn't yet found my passion in women's health. Something was missing. As I began navigating the waters of women's health, I discovered an entire subset of patients who were often marginalized; they were searching for answers and being punted from doctor to doctor without adequate care. These patients suffered in silence for years without getting appropriate answers, and I knew I wanted to dedicate my life to helping them find relief. It was during this time that I decided to pursue my fellowship in urology, focusing my path in medicine on a patient-centered, rather than a problem-centered, approach. That's when I finally found my place.

Understanding the nuances of urological and gynecological pelvic pain, an area of medicine that was essentially untapped, rekindled my passion for medicine. Watching my patients get better and get back to living their lives added fuel to that fire, too. And that, folks, is how I became the Pelvic Pain Doc!

I believe people have the power within themselves to manage and overcome their pain and to regain control of their lives. As I always tell my patients: It's my job to give you the tools to help you treat your-self, but it's how you use those tools that really matters. My goal for this book is to provide you with information not only about helpful treatment strategies, but also to help you gain a well-rounded view of the multifactorial causes of pelvic pain. Armed with the facts, you can begin to take your healing into your own hands.

I also want you to remember that you are not alone in this. Pelvic pain does not discriminate: An estimated 15 percent of people (women and men alike) experience chronic pelvic pain at some point in their lives. In all likelihood, this number is drastically underreported due to social issues like stigmatization, and medical approaches that result in delayed diagnosis or misdiagnosis in many who suffer. This book is for all people, from all walks of life, of all ages and ethnicities, who have been affected by pelvic pain.

Fortunately, great strides have been made in the world of pelvic pain, thanks to clinicians who have pushed boundaries and challenged conventional thinking. Understanding and awareness of causes and treatment strategies for pelvic pain is not enough—knowledge of them must be translated into action to be truly valuable. With lifestyle modifications and active doctor-patient partnerships, this forward momentum will lead to actual lives changed.

And changing lives is what we are here to do. So let's get started!

SECTION 1

UNDERSTANDING THE PROBLEM

1

LET'S TALK BASICS

ELVIC PAIN IS DEFINED as any pain or discomfort, ranging from a sharp jab to a dull ache in the area below your belly button and between your hips that lasts six months or longer. The lower abdomen and pelvic region encompasses all the organs of your reproductive system and most of your digestive and urinary systems. There's a lot happening in the pelvic area—in your stomach, bowel, bladder, uterus, ovaries, prostate, testicles, penis, and more—so the source of pelvic pain can often be tough to identify. See page 200 for illustration.

It is important to consider that pelvic pain mechanisms may involve acute and chronic processes, both peripheral and central to the pelvic area, and may also have a significant emotional component. More often than not, there are multiple "pain generators" at play, which is what can make understanding and treating pelvic pain so complex.

I often hear my patients echo a common belief that a single action will relieve their pain. They might tell me, "When I have my uterus/bladder/vagina/colon/prostate [this list goes on] removed . . . my pain will be relieved." Unfortunately, the solution is not quite as simple as this.

I am reminded of the old Buddhist fable of the three blind men and the elephant. The men conceptualize what the elephant is like by touching it. The first man touched his trunk. "It is a thick snake," he proclaimed. The second reached for his ear. "It is a fan," he said. The third touched his leg. "It is a tree trunk," he exclaimed. Of course, a whole elephant is none of these things. Their error is that of perception: They made dogmatic assumptions based on a limited perspective. The moral of the story is that none of the men were able to take a step back and to see the entire animal.

And herein lies the problem with treating pelvic pain. For the most part, it is never caused by one thing. In turn, this means it is almost never completely treated by a single approach. It is important to constantly reevaluate and use a multidisciplinary plan. If you look at pelvic pain with narrow vision, you are essentially approaching it like the blind men touching the elephant.

COMMON CAUSES OF PELVIC PAIN

Just like there are many diverse symptoms of pelvic pain (including, but not limited to, pressure, burning, painful sex, difficulty sitting, and changes in urinary and bowel patterns), there are many different things that could be causing it. Some conditions are more serious than others. The most serious may require surgical intervention, but most can be treated with various types of medications, in-office procedures, and pelvic floor therapy or psychotherapy (or a combination of any or all of these). If you're experiencing pelvic or bladder pain, the cause could be one of the following conditions:

Vulvodynia or Vestibulodynia: The term *vulvodynia* (chronic vulvar pain) is derived from the combination of the words *vulva* (external genitalia in females) and *Odyne,* the Greek goddess of pain. These conditions are some of the most elusive causes of pelvic pain. Because often there is no obvious cause that is apparent, it can be tricky to get to the root. As a result, patients may suffer for a long time before getting a proper diagnosis. Symptoms of vulvodynia and vestibulodynia include burning or feeling raw in or around the vagina, swelling or throbbing of the vulva, intense itching, and extreme pain during intercourse. A combination of therapies can lead to a pain-free life.

Endometriosis: Endometriosis occurs when tissue *similar* to the uterine lining is found outside the uterus in other parts of the body. This can cause extremely painful and irregular periods, gastrointestinal discomfort, and pain during urination, bowel movements, and intercourse.

Pelvic Floor Dysfunction: Pelvic floor dysfunction refers to a dyssynergia, or an alteration in coordination of the pelvic floor muscles, that can often lead to a change in control over the pelvic floor. With proper pelvic floor function, these muscles assist in normal bodily functions, such as urination and bowel movements. If they become too weak or too tight, a variety of pelvic issues can occur, including pain, incontinence, constipation, and sexual dysfunction.

Interstitial Cystitis: Also known as bladder pain syndrome, interstitial cystitis is characterized by a chronically inflamed bladder. Symptoms are similar to those of a urinary tract infection—such as frequent, painful, and urgent urination, and more specifically pain while the bladder is filling—but without the presence of an infection (negative urine cultures). We believe there may be multiple factors at play, including chronic inflammation that leads to degradation of the GAG layer of the bladder. The GAG layer, also known as the glycosaminoglycan layer, is like the invisible protective coating of the bladder and when degraded (think "holes" similar to "leaky gut") can increase sensitivity and pain. It is unclear if both autoimmune factors and genetics play a role as well. There is data suggesting that neuropathic upregulation (an increase in firing of the nerves) also plays a role and we will delve further into this in Chapter 8. The exact cause continues to be studied, but a multifactorial approach (including medications; various procedures, such as bladder instillations, cystoscopy, and/or certain interventions; and changes to diet and lifestyle) can help to alleviate symptoms.

Prostatitis: For men with pelvic pain, discomfort could be a symptom of prostatitis, an inflammation of the prostate gland. Prostatitis can cause a host of urinary symptoms, such as pain, urgency, hesitancy, or frequency of urination. Men with prostatitis may also experience pain symptoms such as painful ejaculations, or pain in the groin, pelvis, lower back, or testicles.

WHAT'S MORE

Many of these pain generators occur in conjunction with each other. So often, it's not actually a single diagnosis (or a subsequent single medication or treatment regimen, for that matter) that reveals the root cause or provides the answer. The approach I like to take is known as peeling the onion. Taking a nuanced, layered approach to treating pain is key to achieving the desired results. It's the key to understanding and ameliorating root causes. And it is the key to long-term "remission" and prevention.

What's more, pelvic pain is often not just "pelvic pain." It can manifest itself in many different ways.

Some examples:

1. Painful sex
2. Urological symptoms: recurrent UTIs (urinary tract infections), frequency of urination
3. GI (gastrointestinal) symptoms: leaky gut, SIBO (small intestinal bacterial overgrowth)
4. Tailbone pain or pain with sitting
5. Arousal issues and discomfort

Manifestations of pain can occur in many different ways. Your symptoms are your symptoms; they matter, they are often connected, and they can be treated when evaluated with an approach that "peels the onion" to discover the root cause. So let's get started!

2

Behind the Pain: Psychological Distress

Pain has been commonly defined as an "unpleasant sensory and emotional experience associated with actual or potential tissue damage." This definition is provocative, and it opens the door for considering the complexity of pain processing, because it is truly complex. This complexity is what makes pain so hard to understand and treat.

Let's start with the basics. First and foremost, pain is not just a physiological event. In other words, pain is not purely objective: There is a component of perception to pain that makes it "subjective" and therefore more difficult to study, to understand, and to treat. We all perceive pain differently. We have different thresholds for pain and our responses to pain vary greatly.

Let's delve into this a bit further. Living with chronic pelvic pain can be a debilitating, stressful, and all-consuming experience. Pelvic pain isn't something we often talk about with our friends, colleagues, or even family members. Because it can be extremely stigmatized and is not openly discussed, sufferers often feel completely alone. As a result, finding ways to cope can be difficult. As discussed in Chapter 1, sometimes pelvic pain has an identifiable source, such as an infection or cyst. Other times, there are multiple different pain generators. Regardless, discovering the cause can be challenging. All too often, patients are tossed around from doctor to doctor, and meanwhile made to feel that their pain is "all in their head." Well, the truth is that a mind-body connection does exist. Pelvic pain most certainly can be affected by psychological sources. Flippantly dismissing psychological sources for pelvic pain is unfair, unhelpful, and unprofessional.

In reality, understanding the relationship between emotional distress and pelvic pain is one of the most important steps in getting to the root cause. My mission and philosophy of care is to assess and identify the root of what's causing your pelvic pain to help you find relief and regain control of your life. Because there is a cause, even if it is not easily identifiable (more often than not, there are multiple causes or drivers). Here, we'll break down the psychology of pelvic pain and help you understand your symptoms from all angles.

PSYCHOLOGICAL DISTRESS

Often, psychological distress can play a role in symptoms of pelvic pain. Believe it or not, it's the result of the mind-body connection. Past trauma—whether physical, sexual, or emotional—can manifest as pain in the body, which can in turn cause stress, anxiety, depression, and sexual dysfunction, resulting in a cycle of pain and increased symptoms. This cycle takes time to overcome, but relief is possible.

Emotional Aspects of Pelvic Pain

When pelvic pain is caused by an underlying condition such as endometriosis or prostatitis, it is important to be able to assess the primary driver of pain and to "peel the onion" to see what other multifactorial causes may exist. Understanding the science behind pain, and utilizing a multidisciplinary approach, makes it easier for patients to understand where their pain is coming from. Just getting a correct diagnosis can instantly bring a sense of relief for many patients, because it means there's something identifiable that can be treated. But often the cause of pelvic pain is much more difficult to decipher. This can lead to stress, or symptoms of despair and depression, making the entire process of diagnosis and treatment more complicated. Some people suffering from pelvic pain go through months or years of doctor's appointments, tests, and examinations, only to be left with more questions than answers. It can be incredibly frustrating and stressful to live this way. If this sounds familiar, I want you to know you're not alone—and it is not all in your head. Your pain is real, and it is treatable, whether it's coming solely from a physical source or has either psychological or emotional components.

As mentioned, just as pelvic pain can be caused by physical issues, it can also be associated with psychological factors such as stress, past trauma, and abuse. When we go through traumatic experiences, such as physical, emotional, verbal, or sexual abuse, our brains learn to suppress certain emotions in order to protect us from even more harm. If we don't work to resolve our trauma and emotional stress, it can manifest in the body as pain. It's an unconscious response that requires conscious effort to overcome. For example, when Ben was a child he was physically abused by his father. His response to blunt the pain was to clench his jaw. As Ben grew, he developed debilitating headaches particularly triggered by stress. His doctor diagnosed him with tension headaches secondary to temporomandibular joint dysfunction due to his chronic clenching behavior. And this is just one example. Contrary to popular belief, most patients who suffer with chronic pain syndromes don't have a history of abuse or trauma. For patients whose pain does have physiologic causes, trauma work utilizing TMS, CBT, and/or DBT therapies can be incredibly helpful. Please note: A full definition of these terms can be found in the Glossary (page 196).

Breaking the Cycle

In many cases, understanding the relationship and psychology behind or associated with pelvic pain can help put the pain into perspective. The cumbersome process of diagnosing and treating patients with pelvic pain can leave individuals feeling helpless, and this stress and frustration can often present in their symptoms, i.e. manifest physically in the form of pain or discomfort. This leads to an ongoing cycle of pain: The feeling of pelvic pain leads to an increase in (or causes) emotional distress, anxiety, stress, or depression, which leads to an increase in pain symptoms, which in turn leads to further stress and frustration.

Here's how it works: Imagine you broke your leg while skiing a few years ago. As a result, you began to avoid the sport, and even thinking about it makes you tense up. In addition to that, even though your injury is entirely healed, you still experience pain in your leg. This chronic pain isn't actually caused by further injury—it's a message from your brain reminding you of your past trauma. While acute pain (for example, when you accidentally touch a hot stove) protects you from harm, chronic pain can often be related to malfunctioned rewiring that simply gets in the way of living your life. To get back to a life free from pain, you have to break the cycle. The good news is that relief is possible with multidisciplinary intervention. In other words, you have the power to take back control of your body, and with the appropriate tools and support, you can learn to manage and overcome your pelvic pain.

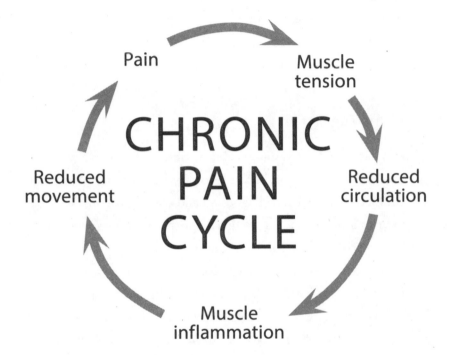

UNDERSTANDING AND FINDING RELIEF FROM PSYCHOLOGICAL RAMIFICATIONS OF PELVIC PAIN

No two cases of pelvic pain are the same. My unique training in gynecological, urological, and neuromuscular causes of pelvic pain has enabled me to understand that pelvic pain looks and feels different for everyone. As such, treatment needs to be customized to your unique situation. The goal is always the same: to give you the tools and resources to understand and overcome both your physical and emotional symptoms. A multidisciplinary approach to treating pain is key. It's important to understand the expertise and additional support that working with a psychologist or psychiatrist can bring. If you feel as though depression, sexual abuse, a troubled relationship, or another stressful situation could be associated with (or worsening) your pelvic pain, speaking to a professional can help you develop strategies to move through it. For treatment to be effective, you need to be open to understanding and addressing the psychological and emotional aspects of pain that are playing a role in your quality of life. It can be tough work, but it's worth the effort so that you can possibly end the constant cycle of pain you've been living with. No one deserves to live with pain. If you're suffering from pelvic pain and notice there are certain emotional or psychological aspects or triggers to your symptoms, it's time to find a physician who understands this association and can help you work through it on multiple levels.

In terms of chronically painful conditions, it is important to understand which various individual factors may have additional negative effects on someone's quality of life. "Quality of life" is an important phrase we use in the field because pain is riddled with subjectivity, and how a patient perceives their quality of life is key for evaluating successful treatment strategies. Specifically, quality of life is not just defined by the ability to complete activities of daily living such as bathing or cooking, it really encompasses the degree to which individuals perceive enjoyment in their lives. For example, if someone suffers from a seemingly simple symptom such as "persistent urinary urgency," it may be so bothersome to them that they can't go to a restaurant to eat.

Limiting the act of socializing potentially effects their quality of life, and also how they view their ultimate progress during treatment.

The goal in such cases is not to replace medical therapy with psychological therapy, but to understand the importance of an integrative approach to understanding and treating pelvic pain conditions.

When considering a psychological perspective of pain, it is presumed that some injury or physiological event, overwhelming patient distress, or a combination of injury and distress causes chronic pain. However, we must remember that physical pain *is real* but that a dual process may be occurring in which both the patient's psychological repercussions to the "stress" of pain and subsequent daily life adjustments are reflected in painful muscle tension and thus greater pain sensitivity. It is when pain moves from acute to chronic (that is, pain that lasts more than three months) that an original physiologic trigger might become less significant while the psychosocial risk factors for pain (specifically anxiety and depression) start to become more pressing.

In other words, the relationship between relatively consistent levels of pain that cause a diminished quality of life is part and parcel with psychological distress (including catastrophizing, depression, and anxiety) in patients who suffer from pain.

When considered together, this body of research clearly begs for a greater exploration and implementation of both psychological and social treatments (lifestyle modifications, dietary changes, appropriate exercises) to complement ongoing biomedical therapeutic management for pelvic pain syndromes. I am convinced by my clinical experience that this integrative approach is key to treatment success and the prevention of recurrent symptoms. In fact, one of the essential purposes of this book is to provide more of you who are suffering from pelvic pain with the tools you need to get started navigating this approach. Who's ready?

3

UNTANGLING THE RESEARCH

S O WHERE DO WE get started?

Part of the reason we are so confused about how to navigate pain syndromes is that the research is hard to conduct: Pain is "subjective," meaning it is part of our personal perception. This subjectivity makes controlled data points difficult to ascertain and therefore difficult to interpret. Ideally, scientists take two groups of people, give them different treatment options for pain (ensuring they don't try any other treatments during this time period), and follow them for 30 plus years. Why can't they try other treatments? Because this can lead to confounding, meaning that the data is skewed because there are too many variables and we don't know what is actually working.

Guess what? That ideal study will never happen. Humans cannot be contained in controlled environments for this amount of sustained time. For this reason, the results of studies for treating pain can never be as definitive as we might like them to be. The key, then, is to draw accurate conclusions by weighing all the evidence about pain from different research areas, from basic science, population studies, and controlled experiments, and then to combine those findings with a touch of evolutionary common sense and context. Easy, right? Wrong. The science of pain is often misunderstood, meaning the research findings themselves are often suspect. This accounts for the kinds of contradictions and misinformation we've seen from scientists and "experts" over the decades.

This is the exact reason that a lot of what is done to treat pelvic pain is considered voodoo by those who don't understand it. Scientific literature in the pelvic pain world is quite limited for a multitude of reasons. Let's start by exploring some of them:

- There are very few randomized controlled trials.
- Most published studies are retrospective reviews.
- There are many dogmatic opinions but little scientific data.
- The tools we have to evaluate responses are often poor because pain is so subjective.
- Pain is multifactorial in nature.

I've said this before and I'll say it again: Treating pain appropriately involves understanding and addressing the concept of multiple pain generators. This makes researching it all the more difficult due to what is known as "confounding" (or as I say, "confusing") factors.

This is important to understand because you will often hear the term "evidence-based medicine" thrown around. I'm not sure everyone who uses it knows exactly what it means, but the approach involves pulling apart the data and applying it to how we treat patients, as a way to ensure safe and effective outcomes. However, both physicians and patients should remember that not all data is created equal. I often joke that being in medicine is like being a part of the debate team, because there are tons of data to support different treatment strategies.

The question we always have to ask ourselves is this: Are the data reliable? Meaning, were there factors involved in how the research was conducted that made certain conclusions essentially less accurate? These are known as biases, and recognizing those biases is important for those who really want to dissect the data. From a patient's perspective, I think numbers and statistics are for the research hall, not the patient room. But, if something doesn't make sense to you—ask! As a clinician and researcher, I always encourage "poking holes" in the data, kind of like a science detective, because this is the only way the field moves forward and we are able to give patients the treatment options that are both warranted and needed.

A BIT MORE ON BIAS

Most research on pain relies on large studies of populations via data that is obtained mostly through questionnaires or recall surveys. Do you remember every single pain or discomfort level you felt this month? How about this week, or even in the last 24 hours? And how do your symptoms fluctuate and change? People often *under-* or *over-* report their symptoms, so questionnaire-based studies tend to "select out" patients whose symptoms may be of a certain severity level that is, in fact, *not* indicative of their long-term or current symptoms. This leads to bias and inaccuracy in the data.

A second point to consider—and physicians, clinicians, and patients are all subject to it—is a phenomena known as confirmation bias. Confirmation bias is the tendency to give greater credence to evidence that fits with our current beliefs. Essentially, we confirm what we want to be true.

Confirmation bias is a concern in sponsored studies. If a study is paid for by a company, the discoveries are far more likely to support that company's product than to question it. In my view, one should always consider who is funding the study. Are there any conflicts of interest? If a study is paid for by a pharmaceutical company or medical device manufacturer, for example, the study's findings may be more likely to support that company's product than to question it. Furthermore, even scientists themselves are sometimes guilty of supporting their preferred theories. They may do so with incredibly dogmatic fervor. As a result, they may believe only the studies that confirm their points of view, essentially cherry-picking the data.

Let's be real. After reading thousands of papers on pain and its causes, even I get confused. But I work to find my way beyond the headlines, apply my understanding of the methods, and objectively analyze the actual data to learn what the studies demonstrate—or equally important, what they don't demonstrate. I've spent hours and hours "nerding out," rummaging through and analyzing data and deciphering all the science so my patients don't have to.

As a doctor, I've also seen, throughout the years, how my patients respond to different treatments and interventions. I have developed a way of treating patients that frees them from the confines of medicine alone and allows them to understand how many factors in their lifestyle, diet, and world play a role in their health. I am curious about what lies beneath our health; I don't receive sponsorship or financial backing from any companies that might have vested interests in the treatment of pelvic pain, nor have I dedicated my practice to proving any particular medical theory or being a proponent of any particular pharmaceutical drug or intervention. I have recommended and overseen all sorts of regimens for tens of thousands of patients over 15 years of medical practice and advocacy. I say this to reinforce how important I believe it is for each patient to receive individualized, tailored care.

My goal as far as this goes is simple: to understand how our lifestyle can and does have an effect on our bodies and symptoms, to discover what we can do to navigate the process of mitigating pain and maintaining wellness with a complete armamentarium, so that we can feel great, live long, and minimize the risks and complications of medications.

And I want the same thing for *you*.

4

BE YOUR OWN ADVOCATE

PELVIC PAIN AFFECTS ONE in every seven women, making it one of the most common women's health issues in the world. As mentioned, pelvic pain doesn't afflict only women. In fact, 1 in 10 men report symptoms. Gender can't and doesn't predict how often or severe someone can experience pain in their pelvis. (Note: While we are using heteronormative terms here, it's important to understand that pelvic pain can affect anyone with a pelvis.)

We have previously touched on how pain, especially at a chronic level, can be associated with downstream psychological challenges that include depression and anxiety. Pelvic pain, and painful sex for that matter, can infiltrate every aspect of a person's life. It can destroy their very sense of being. This is why it's important to understand the tools we have, both at-home remedies and medical treatments, that can help those suffering from pelvic pain to regain control of their lives.

Let's start with a few good pointers on how to get started. First things first: How do you make the most out of your appointment with your doctor? Let's start with some real advice from a real doctor (who tends to be a bit type A and picky, ahem . . . *Who, me?*). I know that a visit to the doctor can oftentimes be a cumbersome process that can leave patients feeling overwhelmed. Add the element of pain to that and it can become a daunting experience. Here's what I suggest:

1. *Preparation is key.* Having access to all prior imaging studies, doctor's notes, tests, and procedures saves a lot of time. And it gives a more accurate picture of procedures and tests that have already been done. As I always say to my patients, "We don't want to reinvent the wheel here." Ultimately, doing the same thing over and over again (that goes for medications, labs, imaging, and procedures) and expecting a different result is Einstein's definition of insanity. *You* are your best advocate, so being well informed of your medical history is paramount to getting the best care that you so deserve.

2. *Keep an open mind.* Oftentimes, we have "researched" our symptoms so much that we walk into a doctor's office expecting a certain diagnosis. When we don't hear what we thought we would, we might stop listening. Guess what, I'm guilty of it as well! But, I will say that as physicians, we have your best interests in mind. (Heck we took an oath promising it, as well!) So, not performing a procedure or not giving out antibiotics or pain meds because we don't deem them necessary isn't to punish anyone. We do our due diligence to examine the risks versus benefits before we prescribe anything. We want to ensure that the care we provide is both effective and safe!

3. *Trust the process.* Treating pain can be a slow process. Pain is multifaceted, and treating it requires a multidisciplinary approach. Understanding that there's no magic pill, and that

the process of uncovering root causes is ultimately the most beneficial aspect of care, can and will help you to keep things in perspective.

4. *As the saying goes, teamwork makes the dream work.* It's important to approach treating pelvic pain as a collaborative partnership. I always tell my patients, "I give suggestions, you make decisions." We are working together to achieve a common goal: It's my job to provide you with options (because there are almost always options), and it's your job to decide what you think will work best for your body and lifestyle. Exact and effective medicine is almost always individualized, meaning there are no set protocols or set next steps. And remember, assessing and addressing root causes takes time. I can prescribe all the medications in the world, but a great deal of success depends on my patients doing their part. Compliance is key.

It's important to utilize the time at your appointments with a full collection of resources. I'm hopeful that some of the tips I provide will enable you to do so. Remember that for women, for issues ranging from constipation and PMS to vulvodynia and pelvic inflammatory disease, there are many gynecological reasons that can cause pelvic pain. Many other urological and gastrointestinal issues can also cause pelvic pain. When pelvic pain flares up, it can be difficult to tell if the cause is a simple condition you can manage at home or if it's something more serious that requires medical treatment. Itching, burning, swelling, fatigue, UTIs, and painful intercourse: It's not a pretty picture, but these are all common symptoms of pelvic pain.

Something that many people don't understand is that pelvic pain is *not* a diagnosis. To be quite clear, the term *pelvic pain* alone means nothing. To find meaning, we must understand the pelvic pain in terms of specific symptoms (such as burning, persistent urgency, painful intercourse), and use that understanding to further decipher exact causes. Where is the pain stemming from? What are the root causes? Even though pelvic pain is extremely common for both women and men, fully understanding the underlying causes requires professional help. Being able to navigate and advocate for yourself in getting that help is the first step to finding relief.

I believe the ability to live the life you want and deserve comes from harnessing all available tools through empowerment and advocacy. Remember that your confusion around pain is not just a personal dilemma. It can impact your family and your community. It can impact your relationships. And it can impact how you view yourself.

Collectively, our lack of education and knowledge about pelvic health issues leads to a great deal of confusion that, in turn, prevents us from actually understanding our bodies. Increasing our education and understanding surrounding these issues empowers us to take control of our own health. And *that* is the first step to gaining back our lives in the midst of pain. And that is one of the biggest goals of this book—to give you the tools you need to take back your life.

This is actually a very exciting time in health care. With every new piece of information, we have an opportunity to better educate ourselves to create healthier lives, healthier people, a healthier planet, and a healthier society. And with every action we take toward better health, we have the opportunity to nourish and heal our bodies. The second section of this book is designed to help you understand each aspect of your pelvic pain symptoms—from their effects on your biology and health to their effects on your mental status and emotions.

Perhaps you might be thinking: Where does my authority on this subject come from? It comes from one place: You. I have seen thousands of incredibly distraught patients become thriving, healthy humans once they took a comprehensive approach to their own health care. Their path toward wellness often involved medications or procedures, but it also incorporated diet, reducing stress, movement, building better relationships, and giving life new meaning.

Let's get to it then.

MEN GET PELVIC PAIN, TOO

In order for men to find relief from male pelvic pain, it's important to first understand what it is. As you now know, pelvic pain refers to any pain originating from the area below the belly button and between the hips. In men, pelvic pain is often labeled as prostatitis. But it's important to understand what this label means and what it lacks. Prostatitis refers to inflammation of the prostate gland, a male reproductive organ that produces fluid and assists in the ejaculation process. Prostatitis is often caused by a bacterial infection, but not always. Prostatitis can affect men of all ages but is more common in men under 50. Prostatitis isn't the only cause of pelvic pain in men, though. Conditions such as nonbacterial chronic pelvic pain, urinary tract infections, sexually transmitted infections, hernias, and gastrointestinal issues may also be at work. The symptoms of male pelvic pain vary in both type and severity, depending on the underlying cause.

Symptoms and Causes of Pelvic Pain in Men

Men with pelvic pain (defined as experiencing pain for anywhere between six weeks and six months) could experience any of the following symptoms, which may stay the same or fluctuate over time:

- Pain or burning during urination
- Hesitancy, urgency, or frequency of urination
- Pain in the abdomen, groin, or lower back
- Pain in the area between the scrotum and rectum (perineum)
- Pain or discomfort in the penis or testicles
- Painful ejaculations

If you're experiencing any of these symptoms of male pelvic pain (especially if this pain does not resolve over weeks or months), you should see a pelvic pain specialist as soon as possible. As previously mentioned, many cases of pelvic pain in men are labeled as prostatitis, an inflammation of the prostate gland. Most of the time, prostatitis is the result of an acute bacterial infection. If the infection doesn't clear after treatment with antibiotics, prostatitis can become recurrent. This is known as chronic bacterial prostatitis. It is also possible to have "prostatitis" without the presence of an infection, often as a result of hypertonic pelvic floor musculature. How so? A hypertonic pelvic floor contains taut bands of muscles that can spasm, causing referred pain or urological symptoms such as frequency or urgency. In other cases, the pain can be caused by a neuropathic upregulation, sometimes derived from nerve damage in the lower urinary tract from surgery or trauma.

Similar to pelvic floor dysfunction in women, this type of male pelvic pain often has no visible cause. This can be frustrating for patients to endure, and difficult for pelvic pain doctors to diagnose and treat. Other potential causes of pelvic pain in men include interstitial cystitis (IC), which is also known as bladder pain syndrome (BPS), irritable bowel syndrome, urinary dysfunction, STIs (sexually transmitted infections), neuromuscular disorders, or psychological triggers, such as trauma or stress. If you're experiencing any symptoms of pelvic pain, it's important you talk to a doctor to get to the root cause and find a treatment plan that's right for you.

Treatment for Pelvic Pain in Men

Living with pelvic pain can be an extremely uncomfortable and stressful experience. But trust me when I say that I do believe that relief is possible for everyone. Through a combination of therapies, I'm confident you can get back to living your life, free from pain or discomfort. Fortunately, most cases of bacterial prostatitis can be treated with antibiotics, as can sexually transmitted infections. Acute bacterial infections typically clear after a single course of antibiotics. Your doctor will choose an appropriate antibiotic based on the type of bacteria causing your infection. However, certain infections can be more difficult to treat. In cases of chronic bacterial prostatitis, you may need intravenous (IV) antibiotics. Treatment length will vary depending on the severity of your symptoms.

If you don't have an infection, your male pelvic pain may be caused by tightness in your pelvic floor muscles. Category IIIB CP/CPPS (chronic prostatitis/chronic pelvic pain syndrome) describes "non-bacterial" prostatitis, often mimicking symptoms of bacterial infections including frequency and urgency of urination, and burning or pain during urination. Pelvic floor therapy can help to release tension in these muscles and help you find relief, as can certain oral medications, suppositories, and lifestyle modifications. If you think your pain may be impacted by psychological distress, consider working with a therapist or psychologist to develop positive coping strategies.

THE ROOT
OF THE PROBLEM

5

Recurrent UTIs or Interstitial Cystitis

I F YOU'VE EVER HAD a urinary tract infection (UTI), you know exactly how uncomfortable, unpleasant, and painful it can be. If you've had recurrent or persistent UTI symptoms with no identifiable infection, you know that it can be frustrating, discouraging, and downright unbearable. This type of bladder pain can often be a sign of a urological condition known as interstitial cystitis (IC), also known as bladder pain syndrome (BPS), due to the discomfort and pain that this condition causes. This is a chronic bladder health issue characterized by pain and/or pressure in the bladder, as well as urinary tract symptoms that last longer than six weeks without an infection present. If any of this is familiar to you, you're not alone. An estimated 4 to 12 million Americans suffer from bladder pain syndrome. Despite its prevalence, this condition is extremely misunderstood and commonly misdiagnosed.

Here are the essential things you need to know about bladder pain symptoms, causes, and treatment options.

INTERSTITIAL CYSTITIS, OR
BLADDER PAIN SYNDROME

The symptoms of interstitial cystitis (IC), also known as bladder pain syndrome (BPS), is very similar to those of a urinary tract infection: bladder pain accompanied by frequent, urgent, and painful urination.

Symptoms and severity vary from person to person, but most people with interstitial cystitis also experience some combination of the following:

- Pressure in the abdomen and/or bladder
- Pain in the abdomen and/or bladder
- Prolonged lower urinary tract symptoms with no infection
- Pain during urination
- Pain during sex
- Frequency and urgency of urination
- Difficulty starting and/or completing a stream
- Pushing or straining to start a stream
- Pain while the bladder is filling

A very important thing to know about bladder pain syndrome is that it is not a urinary tract infection. Although they share many of the same symptoms, they are not the same condition. Their causes are completely different, as are the methods for treating them.

What Causes Interstitial Cystitis?

All too often, interstitial cystitis is misdiagnosed as a UTI. As a result, IC is subsequently treated using antibiotics. But unlike a UTI, interstitial cystitis is not caused by a bacterial infection. At best, antibiotics will not make any difference in relieving symptoms. At worst, they'll create a dangerous antibiotic resistance. Unnecessary antibiotics can lead bacteria to develop "resistances" against overused antibiotics meaning they won't work anymore on that specific strain. This is dangerous because as the bacteria mutate they can become stronger and require IV antibiotics.

Unfortunately, the exact cause of interstitial cystitis is unclear. However, we do have some probable suspects:

- A defect in the lining of the bladder (the GAG layer, also known as the glycosaminoglycan layer, a protective coating of the bladder) that allows substances to penetrate or irritate the bladder
- Neurogenic upregulation, meaning the nerves that travel to the bladder fire more frequently or with increased intensity; this is often related to central sensitization, which is an increase in responsiveness of pain receptors (discussed further in Chapter 8: Getting on Your Nerves)
- Inflammatory issues
- Autoimmune factors in which the body's immune system attacks its own tissues, in this case the bladder

IC is also associated with several risk factors, including:

Other chronic pain syndromes: If you have a condition such as fibromyalgia, irritable bowel syndrome, rheumatoid arthritis, endometriosis, or pelvic floor dysfunction, you may exhibit symptoms of interstitial cystitis.

Gender: Interstitial cystitis is significantly more common in women than in men, although men can still have the condition and may often be underdiagnosed.

Skin and hair color: People with fair skin and red hair are more likely to have interstitial cystitis. (In my opinion, this simply indicates there can be a genetic predisposition, which can be unmasked by other environmental and lifestyle issues.)

Age: Most cases of interstitial cystitis are diagnosed in patients who are in their 30s, but IC is seen in patients as young as 12 and in patients over the age of 65.

Confirmed recurrent UTIs: People who experience reoccurring urinary tract infections are at higher risk for developing IC/BPS. For example, Penelope, who at age 35, had a history of recurrent urinary tract infections that were confirmed by cultures done at her doctor's office and urgent care. During the past year, however, most of her cultures returned negative, although her symptoms wouldn't abate. Ultimately, Penelope was diagnosed with interstitial cystitis and now lives a pain-free life.

HOW DO WE DIAGNOSE INTERSTITIAL CYSTITIS?

A person with interstitial cystitis has the symptoms of a bladder infection, but without the presence of an infection (a negative urine culture). These symptoms include frequency of urination, persistent urgency, or pain (with bladder filling or urination). Diagnosis has become complicated by the emergence of newer technology that can detect lower levels of bacteria. This has led many to question if lower levels of bacteria are related to developing symptoms of interstitial cystitis, but the jury is still out. Back in the day, we (urologists and gynecologists) used to do what was called a potassium sensitivity test. We would place potassium (an aggressive bladder irritant) into the bladders of those who were thought to have IC in order to confirm the diagnosis. How barbaric right? Increasing someone's pain and discomfort to prove that they have a disorder. We've come a long way since then, and we now often confirm our diagnosis with something known as an anesthetic challenge.

An anesthetic challenge is when we place a cocktail of medication into the bladder of a patient in an effort to help coat the bladder's lining and to decrease inflammation. The rationale is this: If we coat an already-inflamed bladder and a patient's pain and symptoms decrease, then by virtue of common sense, the pain must be coming from their bladder. Hence, the cause must be IC/BPS.

Do I Need a Cystoscopy to Diagnose IC/BPS?

First off, what is a cystoscopy? A cystoscopy is a procedure that is often performed in the office in which a urologist or gynecologist utilizes a small camera to look at the urethra (tube going to the bladder) and the bladder. It's commonly used to diagnose issues such as bladder stones, bladder cancer, fistulas, or urethral strictures. People often wonder if this procedure is needed to properly diagnose interstitial cystitis.

The answer is, *not really*. But a cystoscopy can be helpful to discover other conditions (bladder-based lesions, cancer, and so forth.)

A cystoscopy is also helpful to determine if there is the presence of what is known as Hunner's lesions. Approximately 20 percent of patients with IC/BPS have Hunner's lesions. These are discrete areas of inflammation that generally occur in patients over the age of 55. They differ from what are known as glomerulations, or redness of blood vessels, that can occur with the overfilling of the bladder. Patients with Hunner's lesions typically respond to different treatments and strategies than those without Hunner's lesions. Therefore, knowing when they are present is important for care.

HOW IS INTERSTITIAL CYSTITIS TREATED?

Because interstitial cystitis is often misdiagnosed or occurs in conjunction with other pelvic pain syndromes, appropriate diagnosis and treatment can take time. In many cases, you may need to try a number of treatments to find the one that works best to alleviate your symptoms.

Treatment for IC may include any (or a combination) of the following:

- Anti-inflammatory medications
- Tricyclic antidepressants
- Bladder instillations
- Nerve stimulation to block pain and to relax the bladder
- Surgery
- Lifestyle changes, including diet, exercise, and dietary supplements
- Alternative medicine, such as acupuncture
- Pelvic floor physical therapy

We will take a deep dive into both holistic and interventional approaches to treating bladder pain in the third section of this book. But I encourage you to consider taking advantage of one or several of the treatments from the previous list, after a discussion with your personal health care provider. Many can often begin at home.

Living with bladder pain syndrome can be extremely stressful, both physically and emotionally. Relief doesn't happen overnight, but a trusted specialist will help put you on the road to recovery by working with you to assess your condition, create a holistic treatment plan, and support you every step of the way. Remember, the most important step in any health journey is the first one. It's time to start feeling better, one day at a time.

6

When Vaginal Pain Has No Clear Cause

ANYONE WHO HAS SUFFERED from and received treatment for pelvic pain understands the immense relief that comes from getting a diagnosis. If you have spent years searching for answers, finally understanding the underlying cause of your pelvic pain can bring great comfort.

But what if your pelvic pain doesn't have a clear root cause? How do you treat something you can't see? How do you find a health care provider who understands that your pain is real? For many people, finding answers to these questions can feel impossible, especially when it relates to underdiscussed areas like the vagina and vulva.

UNDERSTANDING YOUR ANATOMY

In order to characterize vulvar pain, we need to know and understand the anatomy; there is power in knowing the female anatomy. The main structures of the vulva anterior to posterior (top to bottom) and lateral to medial (out to in) are:

Clitoral prepuce (clitoral hood)

Clitoris

Labia majora

Labia minora

Vulvar vestibule

Urethral opening

Vaginal opening (introitus)

See illustration on page 200.

Pain of the vulva (in general) is known as vulvodynia. Pain iso-lated to the vulvar vestibule is vestibulodynia. The vulva is not the vagina. Most women with vulvodynia or vestibulodynia do *not* have vaginal pain.

- The vulva is the source of the vast majority of sexual plea-sure (not the vagina).
- The vulva is the source of the vast majority of sexual pain (vulvodynia or vestibulodynia).
- Knowing the anatomy of the vulva can help women com-municate better with their partners and health care provid-ers when it comes to sexual pleasure or when something feels off or wrong.

What Is the Vestibule?

The vestibule is a small area of tissue between the inside of the labia minora and the hymenal ring at the opening of the vagina.

The vestibule contains the urethral opening (where the urine exists) and many small glands that produce lubrication (wetness) at the vaginal opening.

The vestibule forms from the endoderm of the urogenital sinus during development (which is a different origin than the vagina or the outside vulva). Because of this, the tissue of the vestibule has different qualities when it comes to hormones and nerve endings. This is important when we discuss treatment strategies.

VULVODYNIA AND VESTIBULODYNIA

Vulvodynia and vestibulodynia are conditions that cause intense, chronic pain in the vulva. It can affect as many as 16 percent of women. This percentage is likely much higher, particularly because it has been estimated that approximately 40 to 49 percent of women with chronic vulvar pain do not seek medical care for their pain. This means estimates are unreliable, and in all likelihood the true prevalence of this condition is dramatically underestimated.

Women with vulvodynia are commonly affected by other chronic pain conditions, such as fibromyalgia, irritable bowel syndrome, temporomandibular disorder, or interstitial cystitis. Collectively these conditions have been termed "comorbid chronic pain conditions" or "chronic overlapping pain conditions." Among women who have such diagnoses, the prevalence rates of vulvodynia are higher than among women who lack any history of chronic pain elsewhere in their bodies.

For some, pain only occurs with contact or pressure, or what we call provoked pain. For others, it's a constant pain that interferes with every aspect of their lives. Vulvodynia is not just a physical condition—it can cause emotional distress, depression, and feelings of hopelessness. Many women suffer with vulvodynia for years before finding a pelvic pain specialist with the knowledge and expertise to diagnose their condition. The key to finding relief from vulvodynia is to first understand the nuances of vaginal pain and then to take a holistic approach to healing.

What Is Vulvodynia and Vestibulodynia?

Life with vulvodynia (or vestibulodynia) is characterized as chronic pain in and around the vulvar area that has no identifiable cause and lasts for at least three months. It can be uncomfortable to sit for even short periods of time, and the pain prevents even the vaguest thought of having sex. Some people may even find it impossible to wear tampons. Vestibulodynia, also known as localized vulvodynia, refers to pain specifically in the entrance of the vagina, or the vestibule. Unfortunately, there is no clear cause of this condition. This uncertainty can make diagnosing vulvodynia or vestibulodynia quite difficult.

Symptoms are similar to other pelvic pain conditions, and they may include:

- Burning sensation in or around the vagina
- Swelling of the vulva
- Extreme pain during intercourse
- Feeling raw in or around the vagina
- Intense itching
- Throbbing of the vulvar area
- Clitoral pain

While often the exact cause is multifactorial, both vulvodynia and vestibulodynia can be associated with:

- Past vaginal infections
- Injury or trauma to the vulvar area
- Hormonal changes
- Allergies or sensitive skin
- Disorders in the pelvic floor
- Neuroproliferative changes (some people have more nerve endings in their vestibule—almost 70 percent more in some cases—making them much more sensitive to things like touch or tight clothing)

For many patients, trying (and failing) to get a proper diagnosis is often the most challenging part of living with vulvodynia. Given the nature of the condition, it can take time for practitioners to understand the underlying cause and to develop an appropriate treatment plan. However, if you're experiencing this type of pain, there is no reason to lose hope. Treatment is absolutely possible.

DIAGNOSING AND TREATING VULVODYNIA OR VESTIBULODYNIA

As we've discussed, vulvodynia and vestibulodynia are tricky conditions to diagnose. Sadly, many patients suffer for long periods of time, unable to get answers for what's causing their pelvic pain. This fact, let alone the intense discomfort, can make life with vulvodynia or vestibulodynia extremely stressful and upsetting.

What to Expect from an Exam?

An in-depth exam is key to diagnosing and treating vulvar health conditions. The full exam has three parts.

The first part of the exam is often the Q-tip test. This procedure, which is used for diagnosing and understanding pain, utilizes a concept known as pain mapping. A cotton swab or Q-tip is used to palpate multiple vulvar and vestibular sites, and the amount of sensitivity or pain reproduced is recorded. Think of the vestibule as a clock. The urethra or urethral opening is at 12 o'clock. The 1 o'clock position is just to the right of the meatus (or urethral opening). The 6 o'clock position is what we call the posterior fourchette. A patient with vulvodynia may have a pain rating of 5 out of 10 at the 2 o'clock position but 10 out of 10 at the 9 o'clock position. It's important that all clock regions are tested. Health care providers may use many variations, but as long as the Q-tip test is reproducible, it's a valid test.

Patients with pain—let's face it, many people—tend to have high levels of anxiety in anticipation of a physical exam when the very point of the exam is to induce that pain. But the more you know about your own anatomy, the more in control you will feel. You can ask your doctor if you can watch what's going on using a handheld mirror during the exam. This can aid not only as an education tool, but it can also help you know the pain is real as you see changes in the skin in this area or visualize reproducibility in pain. In addition, using a mirror allows your doctor to demonstrate how to apply any topicals (as will be discussed in Chapter 11, page 85). This instruction can give you the confidence to do the same in the privacy of your home.

The second part of the exam should include something known as vulvoscopy (examination of the vulva). Vulvoscopy is an examination

---

of the vulva with a special microscope called a colposcope. A colposcope is a large microscope that is used to see the areas of the cervix, vestibule, and vagina to help elucidate any dermatologic changes that may be related to vaginal symptoms. Vulvoscopy itself is not painful, as it is simply a procedure to examine the area and usually lasts no more than 10 minutes. A vulvoscopy is a necessary part of the physical examination for vulvar pain.

It allows us to see:

- Induration (hardening)
- Excoriation (scratches)
- Fissures (small cuts)
- Ulceration (ulcers)
- Erythema (redness)
- Lichenification (skin thickening)
- Hypopigmentation (lighter skin)
- Hyperpigmentation (darker skin)
- Scarring
- Architectural changes (changes to normal vulvar anatomy)

Vulvoscopy helps us diagnose dermatological disorders such as lichen sclerosus or lichen simplex chronicus. It is also helpful in diagnosing vestibulodynia. Redness of the ostia (openings) of the glands of the vulvar vestibule (Bartholin's, Skene's, and greater vestibular glands) may suggest vestibulodynia.

The third part of the exam includes a comprehensive assessment of the pelvic floor. This is done with your doctor, through palpation (touch). In this case, the doctor uses a finger in the vagina to examine all the muscles of the pelvic floor and levator ani complex.

Important muscles evaluated are:

- Pubococcygeus
- Puborectalis
- Iliococcygeus
- Coccygeus
- Transverse perinei
- Bulbospongiosus
- Obturator internus

Followed by an examination of the:

- Bladder
- Compressor urethrae (musculature surrounding the bladder)

HOW IS VULVODYNIA TREATED?

Additionally, it's important for patients and practitioners alike to recognize that vulvodynia can cause more than just physical pain—it can lead to emotional distress, strain on relationships, feelings of isolation, and depression. When treating vulvodynia, it's just as necessary to treat the emotional trauma as it is to treat the physical discomfort. While no single treatment for vulvodynia is effective for every woman, a combination of therapies can lead to a life without pain.

This combination may include:

- Topical medications
- Oral medications

- Biofeedback therapy to train the pelvic floor muscles to relax
- Pelvic floor physical therapy
- Local anesthetics to temporarily relieve pain symptoms
- Psychotherapy to release emotional blockages from past trauma
- Surgical interventions

I cannot stress this enough: Your pain is not in your head. If you're experiencing pelvic pain of any kind, there is a reason. More important, there's a way to find relief.

7

THE PELVIC FLOOR AND
MORE . . . GALORE

THE PELVIC FLOOR ISN'T a part of the body most people often
think about—if they even know what it is at all. But even if you
aren't aware of it, your pelvic floor muscles are involved in many of
your body's day-to-day functions. These muscles assist in urination
and bowel movements, allowing you to have conscious control of your
bladder and bowel. They also provide support for your pelvic organs,
which include the bowel and bladder for men, and the bowel, bladder,
and uterus for women. The pelvic floor muscles play an important role
in sexual health, too. In men, the pelvic floor allows men to achieve
an erection and ejaculation, while for women, voluntary contraction of
the pelvic floor muscles can increase sensation. During pregnancy, the
pelvic floor muscles also provide support to the baby.

But if you don't have control over your pelvic floor, a host of issues
and discomfort can arise. Because the pelvic floor muscles need to be
contracted and relaxed to perform various functions, improper function can cause incontinence, severe constipation, pain during sex, and
more. Fortunately, with pelvic floor physical therapy, you can regain
control of your pelvic floor and get your life back.

———

WHAT IS PELVIC FLOOR DYSFUNCTION?

Your pelvic floor muscles are what you use to control the flow of urine and to make bowel movements. When relaxed, they allow for normal urination and bowel movements—but if they're too relaxed, you may experience incontinence. When taut, they support your internal organs—but if they get too tight, they can cause pelvic pain and gastrointestinal symptoms such as chronic constipation.

In fact, these muscles can get so wound up that even inserting a tampon becomes impossible. This condition, known as hypertonic pelvic floor muscle dysfunction, is caused by tightness in the pelvic floor muscles (the levator ani complex). This area of taut muscle bands can spasm, which decreases blood flow and oxygenation and increases lactic acid, thereby causing intense pelvic pain. This condition is also sometimes known as vaginismus.

Symptoms of hypertonic pelvic floor muscle dysfunction may include:

- Sensations of burning, rawness, throbbing, stabbing, or aching in the vagina
- Urinary symptoms such as frequency, urgency, and incomplete emptying of the bladder
- Pain during intercourse or inability to have penetrative sex
- Hemorrhoids or rectal fissures (tears in the anal area)
- Low back and/or hip pain
- Constipation

There is no one clear cause of pelvic floor dysfunction. Contributing factors for hypertonic pelvic floor dysfunction may include anxiety, stress, hip or low back injury, holding urine, excessive core-strengthening exercises, or physical or psychological trauma. Childbirth, straining during bowel movements, high intensity exercise, obesity, and age may contribute to a weakened pelvic floor.

How Does Pelvic Floor Dysfunction Cause Bladder-Based Symptoms like Frequency and Urgency?

During a normal urination process, when the bladder contracts the pelvic floor relaxes.

However, changes and hypertonicity (taut, often spastic, bands of tissue) within the pelvic floor musculature (namely the muscles surrounding the bladder) often cause a dyssynergia (problems with muscle coordination) where the muscles of the bladder and the muscles of the pelvic floor actually work against each other. When this occurs, the bladder contracts and the pelvic floor actually spasms, often inhibiting complete release of urine from the bladder. Leaving some urine in the bladder can lead to bladder-based symptoms such as the feeling of persistent urgency, frequency, and difficulty starting a stream. Aha!

However, in these cases focusing treatment goals on the bladder won't lead to relief and often leads to the worsening of symptoms. Treating the pelvic floor, however, is part and parcel of addressing the root cause, ultimately allowing the bladder to completely empty and ensuring relief.

As a side note, you should know that pelvic floor dysfunction can occur in any age group. It's not a problem of the old, or the pregnant, just women, or just men. Pelvic floor dysfunction can be universal and important to assess in any patient presenting with pelvic pain.

———

How Does the Pelvic Floor Play a Role in Vulvodynia or Other Pelvic Pain Syndromes?

Let's think of it this way: Acute (short-term or immediate) pain serves a purpose. It alerts us to an issue. Touch a hot stove? The pain signal to the brain causes you to move your hand away from the heat in order to avoid further injury.

Chronic pain, however, is different. It becomes a pattern or cycle that fuels itself. The initial cause often settles into the background, and because it is often no longer the sole reason for pain, the number and type of pain generators change. Pain can also result from the body's attempt to correct for the functional deficits caused by persistent pain, creating compensatory mechanisms that result in imbalances and hypertonicity.

In the same sense, pelvic pain in any form (be it bladder based or vulvar based) can lead to tightening of the pelvic floor muscles through involuntary guarding. Involuntary guarding is a reflexive contraction or spasming of muscles. This tightening reduces blood flow to the muscles and tissue causing a buildup of lactic acid and other inflammatory metabolites, which can and does effect nerve impulses that lead to burning sensations and discomfort. The burning sensation then leads to further guarding and tightening of the muscles, and therein begins the vicious cycle of pain.

I will often say to patients, "What came first, the chicken or the egg?" The truth is that for those who suffer from chronic pain it's often hard to tell. But what I can say with extreme confidence is that focusing treatment on every known pain generator can lead to a complete resolution of symptoms and longevity of symptom relief. There is hope. And a lot of it.

FINDING RELIEF FROM PELVIC FLOOR DYSFUNCTION

Unfortunately, it is often impossible to treat pelvic floor dysfunction until symptoms are already present. Even so, recovery is possible with early detection and intervention. Keeping the pelvic floor lengthened and relaxed is key for strength, balance, and function. Treatment for hypertonic pelvic floor muscle dysfunction, which aims to relax these muscles, may include a combination of techniques.

Your pelvic pain specialist may recommend:

- Pelvic floor physical therapy
- Yoga
- Muscle relaxants
- Warm baths
- Behavioral health approaches
- Trigger point injections
- Botox

Case Study: Barbara

BARBARA made an appointment with my clinic because she was fed up with having to pee two or three times an hour during the day. At age 41, she was finding herself unable to work or take care of her kids in the way she wanted to. In addition, after she urinated she never felt the relief of an empty bladder, saying that, "I feel like I always have to go." As we discussed further, she began to confess that she had recently begun waking up almost three times at night to use the bathroom. In fact, she and her husband had to stop sleeping in the same room because of it. This was further complicated by the fact that their relationship had really taken a hit during the last three years. She had begun to develop pain with sex after her second child, and recently her symptoms of pain with sex seemed to be getting worse, making any type of penetration feel like "knives."

I sat Barbara down and explained to her that we would need to move forward with a comprehensive exam that would evaluate all aspects of her vulva, vagina, and pelvic floor muscles, as the key to bringing her relief would be contingent on evaluating the nuances of her pain. She agreed. Barbara had tried medication and food intervention already. The medicine for overactive bladder seemed to have worsened her symptoms of persistent urgency and her difficulty emptying. Another doctor had diagnosed her with interstitial cystitis and told her to stop all "problematic foods." She was given an extensive list and had in fact gained six pounds on that diet. And by the way, she still had zero relief in her symptoms. Her inability to get relief had started to make her feel depressed and anxious.

The examination showed undiagnosed pelvic floor dysfunction.

Her pelvic floor muscles revealed exquisite hypertonicity (meaning spasticity) and pain when touched. In fact, in sitting down and doing so it was clear her bladder exhibited no pain when palpated during the exam.

Together, we decided that in order to help her get her life back we must proceed with consistent treatment for pelvic floor dysfunction. Her therapy would begin with excellent pelvic floor physical therapy and muscle relaxant suppositories for local relaxation. With that plan, Barbara left my office.

Eight weeks later she came back for a follow-up appointment. She was ecstatic. She could finally sleep through the night. She was now peeing only every two to three hours, meaning she could work and take care of her kids again without feeling attached to the bathroom. She continued to feel pain with intercourse, and while this had improved it had not completely resolved. Another reminder I gave her: "The absence of pain is not pleasure." We continued to work on it all.

Ultimately with more physical therapy and some pelvic floor Botox treatments, Barbara was able to live a pain-free and happy life. She came off all her medications. She is now able to do what I tell all my patients is the definition of relief: "Only call me when you need me." She travels, works, and has pleasurable, pain-free sex!

The secret to her success was in the nuances of a correct diagnosis and treatment. The best markers of success are contingent on healthy, collaborative patient-doctor relationships.

8

GETTING ON YOUR NERVES

O UR NERVES PLAY A vital role in how our bodies function. Without them we wouldn't feel pleasure or pain; we wouldn't be able to sit, pee, or poop. This chapter focuses on the importance of nerves within our pelvis and how much of what we often call an infection or inflammation is actually led by our nervous system. Without getting too technical, I want you to understand that much of our perceptions of pain and discomfort in any area of the body is either regulated or impacted by changes in the nerves. By understanding the role the nervous system plays within the body, you will be able to understand your own triggers and to take steps toward empowering yourself to heal.

Let's start with the infamous pudendal nerve.

WHAT IS THE PUDENDAL NERVE?

For both women and men, the pudendal nerve is the main pelvic nerve that supplies sensation to the lower buttocks, the perineum, and the area around the anus and rectum. For women it innervates the labia, vulva, and clitoris, and in men, the scrotum and penis. It carries autonomic and motor signals from the genitals and anus, and it controls the sphincter muscles that you use when having bowel movements.

The pudendal nerve runs from the lower back (an area known as the sacral spine, segments S2, S3, S4), separates into a right and left branch, which both respectively run along the pelvic floor muscles and then through the pudendal canal (also known as Alcock's canal), where each side divides into three branches.

In essence, the pudendal nerve starts at the bottom of the pelvis, runs to the base of the vagina (or penis), then branches out into three separate nerves that go to the anal/rectal region, the perineum, and the clitoris (or penis).

If any area along this chain from the sacral spine to the end of any of the three branches becomes irritated or injured, we call this pudendal neuralgia.

WHAT IS PUDENDAL NEURALGIA?

Pudendal neuralgia is a damaged, irritated, or trapped pudendal nerve that results in pain. From its location alone, you can see why pain from pudendal nerve damage or irritation would be so disruptive to your everyday activities, not to mention your sex life. Any of the areas it serves can be affected—from the genitals to the buttocks. The difference in symptoms exhibited is dependent upon which part of the nerve is irritated or injured.

Pudendal Neuralgia Symptoms

As you might have gathered, pain is the most common of the pudendal neuralgia symptoms. But the severity of pain can vary from person to person—so can the type of pain: pudendal neuralgia can feel like mild discomfort all the way to a prickling, stabbing, or burning sensation. Some people might even experience numbness. We've had patients describe that their clitoris hurts, or tell us, "It feels like something is in my vagina!"

The onset of pain can be gradual or sudden; it might last for a long time but feel worse sometimes and better at other times.

Specific pudendal neuralgia symptoms include:

- Pain in the clitoris, vulva, perineal area pain, and/or pain in the rectum, especially when sitting (often with the pain on one side being more significant than the other)
- An increased sensitivity to pain—even a light touch or clothing might trigger discomfort
- The feeling of swelling or a foreign object in the perineum or vagina—and only on one side
- Frequent trips to the toilet or the need to urinate suddenly
- Pain during sex
- Difficulty reaching orgasm
- A foreign body sensation in the rectum or perineum
- Worsening symptoms with sitting or with vibration (think long car rides)

What Causes Pudendal Neuralgia?

Of those who have experienced pudendal neuralgia, two-thirds are women. If you've given birth or had a C-section, it's possible that your pelvic pain stems from a damaged pudendal nerve, although it may heal after a few months.

Other causes include:

- A pelvic injury
- Spinning/cycling
- Vaginal birth
- A broken bone in your pelvis
- Pelvic surgery
- Nearby tissue or muscle compressing the nerve
- A tumor—either cancerous or benign—pressing on the nerve
- An infection
- Slipped disk/Tarlov cyst (under current investigation, although there appears to be a loose association)

Activities like prolonged bike riding or horseback riding are known to cause pudendal nerve damage. Or if you've been suffering from years of constipation, this can also affect the pudendal nerve and result in pudendal neuralgia symptoms.

DIAGNOSING PUDENDAL NEURALGIA

It's important for you to share your history and any symptoms with your pelvic pain specialist as soon as possible. You'll be happy to know that the sooner pudendal neuralgia can be identified, the more effective your treatment can and will be.

Be aware that because symptoms of pudendal neuralgia can present similarly to other conditions, misdiagnoses can occur. This sheds light on the importance of having a strong patient-doctor relationship. It also highlights the importance of working with a doctor who has expertise in this area in an effort to determine root causes.

During an appointment your doctor might:

- Press on the pudendal nerve in a vaginal or rectal exam
- Order an MRI scan to see your organs and to reveal if a trapped pudendal nerve is the issue
- Give you a pudendal nerve block—this is an injection given around the nerve to see if your pain decreases or your symptoms improve
- Screen you for possible infections or immune diseases
- Suggest a pelvic floor exam to determine the health of your pelvic floor muscles and to see if skeletal alignment abnormalities exist

TREATING PUDENDAL NEURALGIA

The good news is that pudendal neuralgia symptoms can be alleviated, allowing you to live a life with more comfort and less pain. Lifestyle changes, medication, and physical therapy can go a long way in treating pudendal neuralgia symptoms.

Lifestyle Changes

A good start is avoiding things that make the pain worse—these might be activities like cycling, sitting for too long, or squats. If you've suffered from chronic constipation, then a diet rich in whole grains, veggies, and fruit should help bring your bowels back in balance.

Medication

Both oral and topical medications exist that can help specifically with nerve pain. Your doctor might also recommend injections of a local anesthetic and steroid medication that can alleviate pain for a few months at a time. Botox is another treatment—when injected into the pelvic floor muscles, Botox has been shown to relax muscles that may be irritating the pudendal nerve.

Physical Therapy

A physical therapist will take you through pudendal neuralgia exercises that are designed to help you relax and stretch your pelvic floor muscles, as well as the surrounding muscles that might be irritating the pudendal nerve. The therapist works to release myofascial muscle tension, and sometimes uses trigger point therapy internally through the vagina or rectum. Physical therapy can also help with incontinence if pudendal neuralgia has affected how well you can hold your bladder and bowels.

If pudendal neuralgia exercises in physiotherapy don't help with the pain after 6 to 12 sessions, your pelvic floor specialist might prescribe more serious treatments, such as the following.

Decompression Surgery

When an MRI shows that something is pressing on your pudendal nerve, like a piece of tissue, surgery can move it away from the nerve and reduce your pain. However, surgery is the most invasive treatment for pudendal neuralgia and doesn't always end in success. It also has a lengthy recovery time: from six months to a few years, as nerves heal very slowly.

Nerve Stimulation

For this treatment, a small device is surgically implanted under the skin. The device delivers mild electric impulses to the pudendal nerve. These electrical impulses interrupt pain signals to your brain.

Now that you have a better understanding of the causes, symptoms, and treatment options for pudendal neuralgia, let's take another step in our investigation into the causes of pelvic pain.

WHY IS PAIN SO COMPLEX?

As we know, pelvic pain has a number of different causes, and it may be frustrating to learn that there are no definitive answers as to what causes each symptom or cluster of symptoms. And although we've discussed the multifactorial nature of pain, it's often more complicated than that.

Why is pain so complicated? Why do we struggle to find the help we want and need? Let's delve a bit further into the issue.

The First Biggest Reason: Perception

Pain is a perceived experience, meaning that it is subjective, variable, and open to interpretation. In science, things that can't be studied in a controlled fashion become more difficult to understand. Because pain is subjective, delays in diagnosis and treatment strategies are common. Pain receptors exist throughout our bodies and organs. Some receptors, known as somatic receptors, are directly correlated with the intensity, duration, and location of the inciting stimulus. This is the type of pain many identify as being sharp, pinching, acute pain. Other types of receptors, known as visceral receptors, are associated with symptoms like nausea, bladder pain with filling, and distension. Visceral receptors often have different thresholds, and they can account for pain that is more prolonged and intense. For example, take the symptom of "persistent urgency" in the bladder. This seemingly innocuous symptom can monopolize people's lives and livelihood. The take-home point is this: Pain isn't just pain. Pain can manifest as discomfort, pressure, nausea, or tingling. These, too, are life-altering symptoms, and they are often a result of some sort of neuromuscular cascade. This involves the release of certain neurotransmitters that inevitably cause downstream effects such as increased pain, sensitivity, or involuntary muscle contractions or spasms.

Your symptoms are real.

Your symptoms warrant an evaluation.

Your symptoms can be treated.

It is important to know that pain receptors don't always activate immediately to disrupting stimuli. This can lead to a lag time
between the trigger and the symptom.

Again, it *is* that complicated but it is *not* simply "in your head."
(Although much of pain can and is processed through various por-
tions of our brain.)

The Second Biggest Reason: Pain Is Often Referred

Referred pain is one of the least appreciated mechanisms underlying pelvic pain and other comorbid pain conditions. Referred pain,
or pain that is perceived at one location in the body but actually
occurs in another part of the body, is a regular feature of pain
and can also account for many seemingly enigmatic pain symptoms. Three major questions should be considered when someone
reports pain in a specific location:

1. Is the pain caused by tissue pathology in the target tissue?
2. Is the pain referred from another site exhibiting tissue
   pathology?
3. Is the pain a part of a cycle known as sensory memory or neuromuscular memory?

In practice, pelvic pain rarely fits neatly into existing diagnostic categories, which is not surprising given that vulvodynia, bladder pain syndrome/interstitial cystitis, dysmenorrhea (menstrual
cramps), pelvic girdle pain, and debatably (painful) endometriosis
are often dubbed "diagnoses of exclusion." Therefore, pain assess-
ments based on symptoms, rather than existing diagnostic categories, are useful in deciphering mechanisms of referred pain.
As clinicians, it is important that we all "think outside the box"
when it comes to pain, especially when it seems to be recurrent or

nonresponding. I've found in my own clinical experience that unresolving or recurrent pain is a clear indication of a pain generator that is not being addressed.

The Third Biggest Reason:
Cross Talk! (Yes, Organs Talk)

Do you ever notice that your bowel patterns can affect your urinary symptoms? For example, constipation can increase feelings of urinary frequency, urgency, and sometimes even pain.

This connection is known as viscerovisceral convergence, or cross talk. In practical terms, it means that the neurons converge inputs from different organs in our bodies such as the urinary bladder and colon.

Cross talk establishes three types of functional interactions between different types of neurons:

viscerovisceral (organ to organ)
viscerosomatic (organ to muscle and/or skin)
somatovisceral (muscle and/or skin to organ) interactions

The functional consequence of these interactions is referred pain.

For example, referred deep muscle pain in the pelvic floor muscles can contribute to diffuse (not localized) pain sensations, given that muscle pain can be perceived along the length of the muscle. This pain is thought to result from a neuromuscular reflex that induces painful muscle contractions.

Cross talk that occurs between visceral organs is a key aspect for understanding pelvic pain. Understanding how cross talk works can also be leveraged to facilitate treatment efforts. For example, have you ever wondered why anesthetic blocks sometimes provide only partial relief? Or why treating constipation can help to relieve your bladder pain? It is because successfully treating the pain in one organ can partially alleviate pain symptoms associated with other organs with overlapping nerve innervation.

It drives home the concept of looking at the body as a whole. And while we still have a way to go in understanding more pathophysiology, cross talk is an important concept to keep in mind when evaluating pain.

The take-home point is this: Your symptoms can definitely be related, and understanding this relationship is an important step in receiving appropriate care.

Fourth and Final Reason: Central Sensitization

Central sensitization is a process whereby repeated painful stimulation enhances the firing properties of nerves. Understanding this process is of utmost importance.

There are five reasons for central sensitization:

1. Reduced activation thresholds
2. Enhanced signaling
3. Spontaneous signaling with no stimulus (ectopic discharges)
4. Enhanced signaling with repeated stimulation (wind up)
5. Recruitment of silent receptors that were previously not "pain receptors"

Central sensitization is a powerful idea, as it provides a physiological mechanism for sustained pain in the absence of the precipitating stimulus. Prolonged activation of pain receptors can trigger enhanced activity in spinal cord neurons, leading to increased pain sensitivity. Mind. Blown!

9

ESTROGEN AND TESTOSTERONE AND HORMONES . . . OH MY!

HORMONES. THEY IMPACT US in so many ways. But what role do they have in how pain is experienced? I often hear patients say, "I'm not sure why but my *bladder* pain always increases right before my period." Or, "I notice my symptoms get better during or right after my period." Of course, we can't ignore the fact that menopause often leads to changes in symptoms related to pelvic health, which itself is a subject that could fill volumes. Let's be real: No one book will give you a complete understanding of how your hormones are affecting you—that's what having a trusted doctor-patient relationship is for. Together with your doctor, you can explore the nuances of hormones, and interpret your individual experiences. By understanding some of the basics of hormones in terms of pain, you can be better equipped to work with your doctor. So let's examine some of the basics.

ESTROGEN AND PAIN SIGNALS

Estrogen is implicated in sensation and pain regulation at the peripheral and spinal levels. In the brain, estrogen promotes substances that act like "pain killers," which leads to a decrease in pain signaling to the spinal cord. Believe it or not, estrogen receptors are present in the spinal cord, specifically in the lumbosacral dorsal root ganglia and on peripheral terminals of nerves in the vulva, vagina, uterus, bladder, and ovaries.

Signaling of pain neurons can vary across the cycle as hormones fluctuate. During preovulatory periods of high circulating estrogen, the enhanced structural integrity of tissue allows the tissue to withstand physically rigorous acts of intercourse. In contrast, a decrease or imbalance of female hormones (proven in rat studies!) increases pain hypersensitivity threefold. That's a large number!

MANAGING PAIN PERCEPTION WITH TOPICAL HORMONE TREATMENTS

Let's pause to consider anatomy for a second, because I think there are some aspects that may interest and surprise you. Anatomically, in males the endoderm forms the urethra and male glands (Cowper's glands and gland of Littré). In females, the endoderm forms the vestibule, including the opening of the urethra, and the female glands (Bartholin's glands and greater vestibular glands). As in males, the vestibular tissue in females has many androgen (testosterone) receptors, so the tissue depends upon testosterone to keep it healthy and symptom-free. There is further support for this finding, in that studies have shown that medications that decrease androgens, such as birth control pills, change the tissue of the vestibule, decrease tissue thickness of the labia minora and vaginal opening, and reduce the size of the clitoris after only three months of use. These changes can lead to pain with sex during initial penetration. Studies have shown that these effects are improved or reversed with a topical estrogen and androgen (testosterone) medication applied to the vestibule. There's a power in this combination, for the reasons noted here.

So how does this work? Well, utilizing topical hormone treatment (in the right individualized doses) helps to rebuild the architecture and integrity of the vaginal tissue, thereby normalizing the threshold with which pain receptors in the area are activated. This is an example of the pivotal role that topical hormones play in pain perception localized to the vestibule, which is indicative of its important role in referred and comorbid pelvic pain.

CAN BIRTH CONTROL PILLS
CAUSE VULVODYNIA?

The long-term consequences of oral birth contraceptive use on genito-pelvic pain remain poorly understood. On the one hand, women with estrogen-dependent conditions like endometriosis can benefit from oral contraceptive use. In contrast, extended use of birth control pills, especially low-estrogen formulations, may confer greater risk for developing provoked vulvodynia or vestibulodynia.

Studies have shown that within the vestibule there is an upregulation of pain receptors in women who take birth control pills. We believe that pain hypersensitivity could develop with long-term alteration in estrogen and progesterone levels (altering these levels is how the pills work to prevent ovulation and therefore pregnancy). We also believe this hypersensitivity occurs because these long-term alterations might promote de novo nerve sprouting (the creation of new nerves) and hyperinnervation (a larger amount of nerves than normal).

So why do some women develop these symptoms while others don't?

The answer is genetics. There seems to be a genetic predisposition for certain individuals to experience these symptoms. In particular, the lower amount of free testosterone in these patients (secondary to chronic oral contraceptive use) may confer a higher risk.

HORMONES AND BLADDER PAIN?

Many patients who suffer from IC/BPS (interstitial cystitis, or bladder pain syndrome) report an increase in their pain right *before* their period starts. In terms of the data, there isn't much that confers a hormonal risk factor as a cause. However, what we do know is that as hormones change within our menstrual cycles, so do levels of inflammation. And as levels of inflammation increase, so can bladder pain symptoms.

MENO-WHAT? MENOPAUSE.

Genitourinary symptoms, which affect more than 50 percent of menopausal women, refers to a constellation of symptoms that may be experienced secondary to menopausal changes. These symptoms include vaginal dryness, itching, painful sex (the "genito"), or things such as recurrent urinary tract infections, burning with urination, frequency, and urgency (the "urinary"). Symptoms like dryness, thinning, or changes in the vaginal architecture can lead to changes in the pH of the vagina and alterations in the vaginal microbiome, decreasing the presence of "good bacteria" or lactobacillus. These symptoms have a significant impact on sexual function, daily activities, emotional well-being, body image, and relationships, and yet fewer than 10 percent of symptomatic women are treated with prescription therapy to alleviate their symptoms.

Genitourinary syndrome of menopause (GSM), a condition first defined in 2013, describes the urogenital signs and symptoms many women experience following the onset of menopause. GSM results from the progressive decrease in production of ovarian estrogen and androgen (testosterone). The term GSM was developed to replace the terms vulvovaginal atrophy and atrophic vaginitis, which were outdated because they did not comprehensively reflect the vast majority of symptoms that many women can experience secondary to these changes.

Let's dig in to the why of GSM!

Without estrogens and androgens, over time the vaginal and vulvar tissues drastically thin, and a few key anatomical changes can occur:

- The urethra protrudes and may telescope or prolapse
- The introitus narrows
- The labia minora resorb
- The vaginal pH increases

When these changes occur and the epithelial lining thins, then vascularity, collagen, and elastin decrease, and the smooth muscle structure changes. Resulting symptoms include:

- Decreased lubrication
- Pain with sex
- Urinary frequency and urgency
- Recurrent urinary tract infections

Unlike vasomotor symptoms (hot flashes and night sweats) seen in early menopause, which typically lessen over time, these changes increase in severity over time, and they do not improve without treatment.

In essence, hormones play a pivotal role in our systems and balance. Changes can occur at any age due to many processes. It is important that we clearly evaluate these changes in order to remedy them and to see downstream changes in pelvic and sexual health. Key point: Don't be afraid of hormones!

10

Examining Endometriosis

THE ELUSIVE DIAGNOSIS
OF ENDOMETRIOSIS

M OST OF US NOTICE when something's different about our health. Abdominal or pelvic pain, a shift in your menstrual cycle, pain in other areas of the body. We all know that these can happen for a number of reasons. But what if you're experiencing severe pain or cramping? Trust yourself if your intuition says something's off. Increased pain in the pelvic area or elsewhere can be one of the first signs of endometriosis.

It is important to understand the signs and symptoms of endometriosis. It takes an average of eight years for most patients to receive a correct diagnosis. This statistic is an indicator of the factors that contribute to clinical delays in diagnosis and appropriate treatment.

More recently, there has been a trend to focus on endometriosis as a cause of pelvic pain, and rightfully so given that endometriosis has a history of under- and misdiagnosis. There are entire books focused on endometriosis; however, for the purpose of this book, I would like to help you understand just some basics of endometriosis in the context of the entire body and its interplay with other causes of pelvic pain.

More often than not, endometriosis *does not* act alone. In fact, endometriosis and interstitial cystitis (bladder pain syndrome) are often dubbed the evil twins. A vast majority of endometriosis patients also suffer from other comorbid pelvic pain conditions such as pelvic floor dysfunction, irritable bowel syndrome, neuropathic changes, and vulvodynia. This leads to further misdiagnosis and delays. As a result, pain from these conditions sometimes persists even after appropriate treatment.

I want you to understand that endometriosis can be an elusive diagnosis, but it's one that cannot and should not be missed. This chapter will address the following:

- What endometriosis is
- Initial signs and symptoms
- Possible causes
- Downstream effects
- Treatment
- Prevention

WHAT IS ENDOMETRIOSIS?

Simply put, endometriosis is tissue that is *similar* to the uterine lining and is found outside the uterus in other parts of the body. This tissue goes through the usual process of thickening, breaking down, and shedding like uterine tissue normally would in the uterus. But when this process happens in other organs, the shed tissue doesn't have anywhere to go. So instead of shedding and exiting through your vagina during your period, this endometrial tissue becomes trapped. The presence of these cells where they don't necessarily belong can ignite a potentially severe inflammatory response. This response can lead to wide-ranging symptoms. In the United States, it's thought that about 10 percent of the population can be affected, likely a drastic understatement due to under- and misdiagnosis.

Because endometriosis is tissue that is similar to uterine cells but not exactly, this health issue can occur even when a uterus isn't present in the body. Endometriosis can happen to those without a uterus, to those who don't have periods, and it is not exclusive to women; although extremely rare, it can also occur in men.

If we break it down, there are three types of endometriosis, depending on where it's happening:

Superficial peritoneal lesions: This is the most common type of endometriosis. It's when the endometrial cells grow in the peritoneum—the thin lining of your pelvic cavity.

Endometrioma: This condition happens when endometrial cells form cysts that grow deep in ovaries and can damage healthy ovarian tissue. This type is the most challenging to treat or manage.

Deeply infiltrating endometriosis: This invasive form of endometriosis happens when endometrium grows under the peritoneum—near or on other organs like your bowels or bladder; 1 to 5 percent of women with endometriosis have this kind. It is often challenging to treat.

FIRST SIGNS OF ENDOMETRIOSIS PRESENTATION

An unusually painful menstruation is not the only symptom of endometriosis. Some don't experience this telltale sign at all. And at times, the level of pain depends on where the uterine-like tissue is growing and how much of it is present. So with that in mind, consider if you have these other early symptoms of endometriosis:

- Pain when urinating or having a bowel movement
- Blood in your urine or stools
- Pain during or after sex
- Excessive bleeding during your period
- Excessive bleeding between your periods
- Back pain during your period
- Gastrointestinal issues such as diarrhea, constipation, nausea, or bloating
- Nausea or vomiting
- Difficulty getting pregnant
- Fatigue

An examination can also uncover the possibility that your symptoms are because of another issue, or perhaps a concurrent one. Endometriosis can sometimes be confused with irritable bowel syndrome (IBS), pelvic inflammatory disease (PID), or ovarian cysts.

WHAT CAUSES ENDOMETRIOSIS?

The exact causes of endometriosis are still unknown, but some theories (although controversial) are as follows.

Genetic factors: If a first-degree relative such as your mother, sibling, aunt, or grandmother via either the maternal or paternal line has had endometriosis, there is a seven- to tenfold greater chance of developing endometriosis.

Environmental factors: Studies show that 9 percent of female fetuses have endometriosis. While this may be inherited (a genetic factor), there is also data suggesting exposure to dioxins can increase the risk of developing endometriosis. Dioxins are highly toxic compounds found in by-products of household and gardening products. If a mother is exposed to dioxins while pregnant, her fetus may be exposed to these damaging effects as well.

Retrograde menstruation: It's possible that menstrual blood flows back into the fallopian tubes instead of out the vagina during menstruation. In this case, endometrial cells stick to your pelvic walls and possibly other pelvic organs where they grow, thicken, and bleed over many menstrual cycles. While some still hold this view, it has fallen out of vogue, as it is somewhat myopic to view a complex condition as being caused solely by menstrual blood flowing back into the fallopian tubes; however, it is a theory that exists, nonetheless.

Cell transformations: With this, two possibilities exist. One possibility is that hormones change peritoneal cells—the cells that line your abdomen's inner side—into endometrial cells. The other possibility is that hormones or immune disorders transform embryonic cells into endometrial cells during puberty.

Lymphatic system transport: This is when blood vessels or your lymphatic system carry endometrial cells to other parts of your body.

Immune system disorders: With a compromised immune system, it's possible that endometrium cells end up growing in abnormal places. That, or your body can't recognize this endometrial tissue and so won't begin to attack it.

Scar tissue: If you've had major pelvic surgery like a C-section or hysterectomy, endometrial cells can implant themselves into the scar tissue or leak out of the scar tissue into the pelvic cavity.

DOWNSTREAM EFFECTS OF ENDOMETRIOSIS

If you know someone who has endometriosis, you might have witnessed how incredibly difficult it is for them, and how much it affects their quality of life. As with many health conditions, endometriosis can lead to other complications, such as the following.

Ovarian cysts: Cysts can form when endometrial tissue has made its way to the ovaries.

Scarring within organs: Endometriosis can cause inflammation in the affected organs. Your body responds to the inflammation by forming scar tissue during the healing process. This scarring can prevent blood flow to the surrounding tissue.

Infertility: About one-third of those with endometriosis can have difficulty getting pregnant. Endometriosis can affect fertility in two ways: It can block the fallopian tube and prevent an egg and sperm from uniting; and less commonly, the tissue can directly damage the sperm or egg.

Cancer: If you have endometriosis, the risk of ovarian cancer is higher but is still relatively low. Even more rare is endometriosis-associated adenocarcinoma, which is cancer in the glandular organs and can happen later in life.

Mental health effects: It goes without saying that endometriosis and its possible effects can challenge your mental health; some women experience depression or anxiety because of it. Unlike many other medical conditions, the pain of endometriosis does not always progress in incremental steps, meaning the progression of disease isn't always correlated with pain level. Someone with stage I endometriosis can have a level 12 out of 10 pain. The potential of being in pain on average of eight years, without answers, a plan, or resolution, can absolutely play a role in a patient's mental health. We have to do better.

HOW TO TREAT ENDOMETRIOSIS

Let's get to the million-dollar question: Does endometriosis have a cure? A complete endometriosis cure hasn't arrived yet, but, thankfully, there are options for minimizing its symptoms and managing its effects. So, with treatment, it's definitely possible to have endometriosis and go about your life with minimal disruption. One of the most important aspects is early diagnosis and an understanding of any other pain generators that may be present.

Treatments range from over-the-counter pain medications and at-home care for mild symptoms, to hormone therapy, contraceptives, or prescription medications and surgical interventions that include excision, ablation, or hysterectomy.

HOW DO I PREVENT ENDOMETRIOSIS?

Unfortunately, you can't fully prevent endometriosis, at least as best we know at this point. But if you start noticing early signs of endometriosis, what you *can* do is work toward lowering your estrogen levels. Higher estrogen levels have been linked with the signs and symptoms of endometriosis.

Some prevention options include:

- Birth control medication: Contraception like pills, patches, or rings help regulate estrogen levels.
- Regular exercise at least four times a week: Lowering your body fat contributes to lowering your estrogen levels.
- Avoiding large quantities of alcohol: A suggested guideline is no more than one drink a day.
- Avoiding large quantities of caffeine: Studies have shown that more than one caffeinated drink a day can increase your

estrogen levels. It's surprising, but even a soda or green tea has enough caffeine to affect your estrogen levels.

- Making overall changes to your diet: Try doing things such as upping your omega-3s, reducing your trans fats intake, eating lots of fruits and veggies, and reducing red meat. Fill up on legumes and whole grains, too.

The biggest thing I want you to be aware of is that, more often than not, endometriosis doesn't act alone. There are often multiple different pain generators occurring at the same time in the form of interstitial cystitis, pelvic floor dysfunction, central sensitization, IBS, pudendal neuralgia, and vulvodynia and/or vestibulodynia. It's important to have all pain generators evaluated in order to receive optimal care and symptom relief. Endometriosis is not an all-encompassing term, and while it has become an increasingly popular diagnosis, I implore you to understand its ramifications in conjunction with other causes of pelvic pain. This is the best way to obtain complete symptom relief in the setting of complex diagnoses.

Case Study: Caitlynn

CAITLYNN initially came to me for a long-standing history of debilitating periods. She was 42 years old, but this problem had been occurring since she first got her period at age 12. Her periods would be so painful and heavy that she would almost always stay home from school because of it. Even though Caitlynn's mother was a pediatrician, Caitlynn and her mother really hadn't explored a diagnosis for her condition. She had gotten pregnant easily with her first child, but her issues really magnified after she gave birth. She noticed the urinary frequency that developed while she was pregnant with her firstborn never resolved. In fact it worsened, as did her feeling of pain with bladder filling, which was particularly debilitating immediately prior to starting her period.

Her OB-GYN had recommended restarting birth control pills, but Caitlynn was hoping to get pregnant again soon with a second child, so that didn't make sense to her. This was compounded by the fact that she and her partner had been trying to conceive for more than six months and her symptoms of bladder pain and frequency seemed to be worsening.

She admitted that she couldn't imagine living like this much longer, "Especially when I'm pregnant. What is going on?"

Caitlynn and I had a long discussion. Her bladder was exquisitely tender on exam. She told me she had started having trouble eating pizza and tomato sauce, as she felt her symptoms extremely heightened after this. But she was also anxious to get pregnant, as she felt she "wasn't getting any younger."

We decided the best thing to do was take a stepwise approach to her treatment. I recommended her to a highly regarded endometriosis specialist with expertise in infertility, who wound up recommending resection surgery for endometriosis after a complete evaluation.

It was clear that Caitlynn in fact had a double whammy: the "evil twins" of both endometriosis and interstitial cystitis. We placed her on a low-dose anti-inflammatory and performed six to eight bladder instillations to recoat the bladder simultaneously.

Soon after, I received a birth announcement for Caitlynn's second child. She did really well after treatment. She still wants to come in for maintenance for her bladder pain symptoms after eight weeks or so. She's a prime example of looking at our bodies as a whole and finding treatments based on root causes to achieve the best results.

SECTION 3

TREATMENTS

11

MEDICATIONS

TREATMENT OPTIONS FOR PELVIC pain have evolved with our understanding of human anatomy and function. In ancient times, pain therapies were, for the most part, limited to the treatment of symptoms with little knowledge of underlying causes. Then, the late 19th and early 20th centuries saw a surge in medical knowledge and gadgets, and with this came the notion that pain *must* have an obvious source that could be identified with modern technology. When it became clear that pain was harder and harder to identify and distinguish regardless of the additional knowledge and technology, many chalked it up to psychosomatic causes, meaning "It must be in their heads."

I like to think that this archaic philosophy is a thing of the past. I would say that strides have been made within the past 15 years with the development of patient support groups and dedicated medical organizations, often working collaboratively. Interdisciplinary therapy and research projects are currently underway. Efforts have been expanded to define the causes of pain that we currently know exist, with the goal of developing targeted and personalized therapeutic approaches. This momentum can and should be translated to patient care as well, with patients being given the tools to understand the causes and treatment options for their pain. And this chapter will attempt to do just that.

Let's start with medications. A plethora of medications are often used to treat symptoms of pelvic pain, and your health care provider's specific plan for you may include some of these. Some of the most common are various types of antidepressant medications. What I always tell patients is that while we often use various antidepressants to treat pain, we don't necessarily use them in "antidepressant" doses. In other words, we tend to use them in much lower doses, the goal often being to downregulate the nerves reaching the pelvis.

The biggest questions I get in regard to oral medication for pelvic pain is, "How long do I have to be on this medication? Will it fix the issue or just mask it?" The answers are complicated. Although I never want patients to become dependent on a medication, there are instances within our health care journeys that require a "raft": some help to get us to the next place. Medications can help "decrease the volume" of pain so we can make sense of all the noise. It's always important to understand the risk-benefit ratio of all medications. And the best way to do that is to have a frank discussion with your physician about their philosophy. You want to make sure it is in line with yours.

ORAL MEDICATIONS

Antidepressants

One of the most common antidepressants is amitriptyline (Elavil), which is a tricyclic antidepressant (TCA). It has become a staple of oral treatment of IC/BPS (interstitial cystitis, or bladder pain syndrome). Amitriptyline to manage IC/BPS is used off-label; however, clinical experience and data from trials support its use. Off-label use of medications is quite common in the pelvic pain field. By definition, "off-label" usage is simply using a medication for a condition that it has not officially been approved to treat. So amitriptyline, while falling into the category of a TCA, its "on label" use is for depression; when used at lower dosages it is particularly helpful for treatment of symptoms related to interstitial cystitis.

The American Urological Association guideline graded the strength of evidence as Grade B, meaning that research used randomized controlled trials (RCTs) as a basis of effectiveness. Despite the promise of this medication, like everything in medicine we must weigh the risk-benefit ratio when considering TCAs.

This brings up an important question: Why do TCAs even work?

- Anticholinergic properties. In straightforward terms, this drug inhibits the action of a chemical messenger. For this reason, this medication can help with bladder-based symptoms such as urinary frequency and urgency because it decreases how often the bladder contracts. Think of the bladder as a muscle, less contraction equals less urgency and frequency.

- Blocks reuptake of serotonin and norepinephrine, the neurotransmitters involved in pain. "Blocking reuptake" increases neurotransmitter availability in the central nervous system, which can be helpful in relieving pain.
- Antihistamine effect. We believe one contribution to the onset of IC/BPS may be the presence of chronic inflammatory cytokines, leading to the degradation in the GAG layer. Antihistamines block the release of inflammatory cytokines by mast cells in the bodies (the cells recruited during times of inflammation).
- Sedative effects. Using TCAs for some pelvic conditions is an instance when the side effects of an antidepressant become beneficial. Many providers often instruct patients to take antidepressants at night, and while they can make you quite sleepy, this side effect is actually beneficial in helping those who suffer from nocturia, which is frequent nighttime waking to urinate.

Keep in mind that for most medications to have a therapeutic effect, meaning for them to actually work, they must be used at appropriate doses. This oftentimes becomes impossible for some patients, due to their inability to tolerate these medications at certain doses.

A percentage of people will experience some side effects with this medication:

- Fatigue (45%)
- Constipation (42%)
- Dry mouth (42%)
- Dizziness (33%)
- Headache (32%)

Amitriptyline and other TCAs such as nortriptyline have also been used to treat generalized vulvodynia. The mechanism behind this involves its effect on serotonin, norepinephrine, and its effect on histamine receptors and sodium channels.

Gabapentin

Gabapentin is one of the most studied and utilized medicines for managing pain. When used for appropriate reasons (such as treating neuropathic pain related to IC/BPS, pudendal neuralgia, and vulvodynia), the efficacy of gabapentin is anywhere between 50 and 82 percent, which is quite significant.

Think of gabapentin as a good tool for "decreasing the volume" of the pain. While gabapentin falls into the category of an anticonvulsant, don't let this categorization scare you. Gabapentin essentially acts through neural pathways in the brain to alter messages and excitement using chemical substances (neurotransmitters) in the brain. Specifically, it is thought to work on calcium channels to block the release of glutamate and substance P.

Decreasing the volume of pain is helpful in patients whose pain may be cycling. I find gabapentin to be most helpful when used in combination with other treatment strategies such as muscle relaxers or topical medications (depending on the specific diagnoses at play). I try to steer clear from placing patients on medications as a long-term treatment strategy, as I think it hinders understanding, evaluation, and treatment of root cause(s).

Side effects of gabapentin are very similar to the side effects of the TCAs previously discussed. And gabapentin's side effects are generally dose dependent (doses range from 100 mg to 3600 mg):

- Fatigue
- Constipation
- Dry mouth
- Dizziness
- Headache

Muscle Relaxers

Muscle relaxers can be very helpful for patients who have hypertonic pelvic floor dysfunction. They can be taken both orally or as suppositories, and they work to help keep the muscles of the pelvic floor relaxed. When used correctly, muscle relaxers can help patients decrease the frequency, urgency, and difficulty of starting a urinary stream.

Muscle relaxers come by many different names, such as:

- Diazepam
- Cyclobenzaprine
- Methocarbamol
- Baclofen

Many prefer to take their muscle relaxants in suppository form, which has fewer side effects than the oral form. When taken orally the most common side effect encountered is tiredness or lethargy. This is why the advent of muscle relaxers in suppository form has been particularly helpful to those suffering from pelvic floor pain and dysfunction. Utilizing muscle relaxers in a suppository form offers localized neuromuscular relaxation without the often debilitating side effects. These suppositories can be placed rectally or vaginally. There is some data to suggest that rectal absorption is superior to vaginal; however, this varies on a case-by-case basis. I often suggest that patients try it rectally or vaginally (for vagina owners) to see which works best for them.

Antihistamines

Hydroxyzine is medication that falls under the category of a first-generation histamine-1 receptor antagonist, similar to how you may think of anti-allergy medications like Benadryl. Inflammation is often thought to be a key component of pelvic pain syndromes. And inflammation often causes the cycle of pain, which makes diagnosis and treatment exceedingly difficult. In open-label studies (where both researchers and participants know which treatment is being administered, i.e. no one is "blinded), anywhere from 25 to 75 mg of hydroxyzine was shown to reduce symptoms of nocturia and bladder pain in patients with IC/BPS. Many practitioners also prescribe this medication for patients with inflammatory vestibulodynia, although this is an off-label use. The most prominent side effect of this medication is sedation or lethargy. Utilizing antihistamines at night can take advantage of these sedative properties to enhance sleep while retaining its antihistaminic actions during waking hours. Win-win if you ask me!

Oral medications can be utilized as an excellent step toward relief from pelvic pain. But there is often much more that can be done. On that note, let's keep going!

TOPICAL MEDICATIONS

Topical treatments are commonly used in the treatment of pelvic pain, specifically from the subset arising in the vulva. The nice thing about topical medications is that they can be used as a first line of treatment, or in conjunction with oral medications or other treatments. Topical medications are often prepared in a base, and that base is important for how the active component is absorbed. Unfortunately, the base can also be an irritant. This means that working with a reliable compounding pharmacy and a knowledgeable physician is key. One of the biggest benefits of compounding medications into a topical form is that side effects are decreased. This is due to decreased levels of systemic absorption. The downside is that it often takes time (in the way of 8 to 12 weeks) to start seeing drastic changes.

All the medications we discussed in oral form can come in topical concoctions. This is important for a multitude of reasons, namely a decrease in systemic absorption, which means little to no side effects! However, the application of any topical agent to the vulva and vestibule must be done with care so as to avoid irritating sensitive tissue. Localized burning can sometimes occur and last up to two weeks, which highlights the importance of working with a trusted compounding pharmacy. In my opinion, a knowledgeable compounding pharmacist is one of the most important parts to the team approach for treating patients. You can count on a trusted compounding pharmacy to suggest hypoallergenic bases for creams and ointments, and to avoid ingredients that may exacerbate symptoms, creating a topical medication that can still achieve maximum therapeutic effects.

It is important to tease out absorption patterns for greater efficacy, and to remove additives that may cause irritation. The goal is to create an individual, localized topical medication. When done correctly, it is life altering!

Hormones

All vaginal pain cannot simply be treated with topical hormone medications, because not all patients respond to them. In terms of understanding the physiology of how hormones work in the vestibule, one must understand that the vestibule contains both estrogen and androgen (testosterone) receptors. This variance in receptors is often a reason why localized, estrogen-only topical medications don't always produce the desired effects.

Localized Applications of Estrogen

Creams and Ointments: These applications are the most common forms of localized estradiol (estrogen) preparations. One of the biggest benefits to this form of treatment is that they are generally well tolerated, and they are covered by most insurances. Studies looking at localized estradiol in patients with genitourinary symptoms of menopause show that it can help prevent urinary tract infections and help with lubrication and pain during intercourse.

Suppositories: Estradiol suppositories work similarly to the equivalent creams and ointments. The benefit of any and all of these localized estradiol preparations are low systemic absorption (thereby decreasing side effects) and localized benefits.

Estradiol and Testosterone: The combination of estradiol (estrogen) and testosterone is a powerful one. Recent data suggests that there are almost 70 percent more androgen (testosterone) receptors than there are estradiol (estrogen) receptors. Not saturating or ensuring that both estrogen and testosterone receptors are bound by the correct hormones can often render estradiol-alone preparations less effective. I like this preparation (a combination of both estradiol and testosterone) because it combines both of these hormones, and it can be delivered in a very soothing base. This can be a godsend for those who have significant atrophy or pain. The only major downside of this preparation is that it must be made in conjunction with a compounding pharmacy, and because the data on its efficacy is "newer," it is often not fully covered by insurances. However, this is often a small price to pay for greater relief and benefit. It is like I always say, "It's like me having a tennis racquet and Roger Federer having a tennis racquet: We both play tennis, but he plays a lot better than I do—we both have the same tools, it's just how we use them." Put another way: The secret in the sauce is often in the nuances of the ingredients.

Gabapentin

Topical forms of gabapentin come in different percentages (2 to 10%). Topical preparations of gabapentin have been used in the treatment of vulvodynia (both localized and generalized) with good tolerability and a low incidence of systemic side effects. One interesting study showed that 80 percent of patients who utilized topical preparations of gabapentin had anywhere between 50 and 100 percent improvement.

Topical gabapentin works similarly as the oral form. Essentially it is used to downregulate the firing of the nerves, which can be thought of as "decreasing the volume" of the pain. The difference is that topical gabapentin can decrease localized inflammation and allow for long-lasting desensitization. Now, don't get nervous. Often, when I use this phrase in the office, patients worry. "Will I be numb?" they ask. "Will I lose my ability to feel anything down there?" The answer: No. Topical gabapentin works well in patients with a localized neuropathic or neuroproliferative component to their pain. So while it downregulates the nerves, it does not completely numb them or make them dysfunctional.

Again, this treatment decreases a "loud volume" of pain, so the pain comes through at a more "normal," well-tolerated volume.

Amitriptyline-Based Preparations

The use of topical amitriptyline is a preferable alternative to those who wish to avoid the annoying side effects often caused by oral tricyclic antidepressants. These side effects include fatigue, weight gain, constipation, and dry mouth. The topical use of amitriptyline is not as well studied as gabapentin topically; however, it does also come in different preparations and dosages, and anyone in the field who has been doing this for a while can tell you there is an absolute anecdotal benefit.

Different preparations include:

- Amitriptyline 2%
- Amitriptyline 2%/baclofen 2%
- Amitriptyline 2%/ketamine 0.5 to 2%

Much of the controversy and difficulty in the field of pelvic pain lies in the paucity of research. This lack of research is due to difficulties in diagnosis and the subjectivity of pain, especially in areas of the body that are stigmatized and often not openly discussed. What I love about topicals is that I can titrate (incrementally alter; see page xxx) medication dosages and compound certain medications together based on the nuances of individualized symptoms and exams. It demonstrates that medicine really is a combination of science and an art. To better determine which compounds may be right for you, I definitely suggest you make an appointment with a specialist who commonly prescribes and understands how to appropriately dispense these medications. I give you these options of medications, and the pros and cons, so you can appropriately discuss and understand these interventions. It is important to me that this book provide you with the knowledge you need to be your own advocate and empower you to seek the care you need. I firmly believe healing is possible—I've seen it with my own patients.

Cromolyn

Cromolyn falls in a category of medication known as mast cell inhibitors. Topical forms of this medication stop the release of inflammatory cytokines often involved in symptoms of redness, itchiness, and burning. In studies to determine its effectivity, 53.8 percent had at least 50 percent symptomatic improvement. I find this compound to be particularly helpful in those patients who have a great deal of "itching" without an apparent dermatologic cause, such as lichen sclerosus or lichen planus (see page 198).

PERFORMING YOUR OWN VULVAR EXAM!

First off, if you have any concerns about the vulva, it is always best to see a gynecologist, nurse midwife, or clinician who is experienced in women's health. However, we *must* all know our own bodies and be well versed in what feels and looks normal for *us*, which is not a universal thing.

I suggest taking a handheld mirror and having a look. Let's start.

- **Anatomy:** Know thyself, as I always say. Notice the size and shape of the clitoral hood, clitoris, labia majora, and labia minora. Notice any changes such as fusion (or sticking together of tissue) or resorption (visualized shrinking of the skin or thinning).
- **Discoloration:** Take a look at the skin of the vulva. Do you notice lightening, darkening, or redness of the skin? Depending on the exact location, this can be normal or a sign of dermatologic change, infection, or inflammation that leads to architectural changes.
- **Texture:** This is a *big* one. Do you notice any thickening or thinning of the skin? This can occur as a side effect from taking medications, or it can be caused by inflammation. It can be related to pH changes in the tissue that are often compounded by infection. This condition can be extremely bothersome, and it absolutely warrants further evaluation!
- **Bumps:** Listen, some bumps are normal and some bumps are not. The most common condition with "bumps" is known as folliculitis. These are "razor bumps," or ingrown hairs, that can develop inflammation and sometimes infection. Another cause is a sebaceous cyst, which is a flesh-colored, painless bump. A Bartholin's cyst can be present as well and would be found as a bump at the bottom on the vaginal opening.

Infectious causes of "bumps" can include genital warts, which are painless, flesh-colored, cauliflower-like bumps, and herpes, which would appear as a small cluster of blisters. Bumps in general have a wide number of causes; however, it is always important to rule out things such as vulvar cancer, especially when and if a bump is constantly irritated and does not resolve with treatment.

Performing a self-exam is key, especially when you sense things are awry but have difficulty finding an explanation.

Lidocaine

Lidocaine is what I also like to refer to as a "raft," a tool to help some patients get to the next place. Lidocaine is not a medication that will alter root causes; however, some patients find it helpful when used on an as-needed basis, often prior to inserting tampons or penetrative intercourse. Lidocaine is not recommended as a first-line treatment for vaginal or sexual pain, but it can be used as a tool to manage pain that is extremely unbearable. Topical lidocaine can be used in a 2% form (often over the counter or via prescription at local pharmacies) or a 5% form. While the 5% form is stronger, it can cause increased burning, especially when initially placed.

In instances when someone needs lidocaine but it burns them too much when placed, it can be compounded with soothing bases such as aloe vera (to cool) or coconut oil to help minimize its initial irritation.

Let me clear: Lidocaine can be helpful, but it cannot and will not be helpful in the long-term analysis or treatment of root causes of pelvic pain syndromes, including vulvodynia or pudendal neuralgia.

Capsaicin

Capsaicin, which is often used as a last resort, is a topical medication that helps to produce a desensitization to burning and so decreases pain. It is thought to act on vanilloid receptors, which are peripheral terminals of pain neurons. In studies conducted on patients with neuroproliferative vestibulodynia, it is thought to be a helpful alternative to those who may have previously undergone surgery (vestibulectomy) but experienced returned pain, or for those wishing to forgo surgery. It should be noted that there is a great deal of burning with topical applications of capsaicin, often rendering it difficult for some patients to comply with it. I always recommend patients discuss this option fully with their providers, and that they work with a provider who has done this protocol many times before. Due to the severity of burning that can occur, in addition I would recommend an in-office trial and a slow titration up for the duration of application.

As you can see, there are many different topical agents that can be used for the treatment and management of pain. It is important for you to work with a trusted provider to come up with the best medications for you. Ultimately, I think it is important for you to know that if oral medications don't work well for you, there are other options that can be just as effective, if not more effective, with fewer side effects.

BLADDER INSTILLATIONS

What the heck is an instillation? And you're going to put that where? Let's get a bit scientific here. Bladder coating agents are commonly used to treat interstitial cystitis (IC), or bladder pain syndrome (BPS). These agents are thought to address epithelial dysfunction. Epithelial dysfunction is a degradation in a microscopic layer of the bladder known as the glycosaminoglycan layer (GAG layer). This layer is thought to protect the bladder, and degradation of it is thought to be one of the causes of IC/BPS.

Think of wearing a raincoat. If your raincoat has holes in it, won't you feel the rain more? It can bother you, right?

In the same respect, a degradation in the GAG layer can allow the bladder wall to be irritated by urinary substances, resulting in a sequence of events that include recruitment of inflammatory cells, mast cell degranulation (a cellular process that releases cytokines or molecules that can increase inflammation), and neurogenic inflammation. Over time, chronic inflammatory processes and neural activation lead to an increase in local nerve growth factors, nerve ingrowth, and neural sensitization. So the concept of essentially placing a medication (or cocktail of medications in this case) into the bladder to recoat this area, almost acting as a varnish, would appear to be a logical approach to addressing a primary pathophysiological factor in IC/BPS.

How is this done?

Recoating the bladder can be attempted in multiple ways. One of the most common is to directly place the medication into the bladder via a catheter. The good news is that the catheter does not stay in place. It is simply used as a vessel to place the medication cocktail containing "recoating" agents into the exact area needed. However, the efficacy of this treatment is not immediate, as it takes time for the bladder to heal.

An oral medication known as pentosan polysulfate (actually the first and only FDA-approved oral medication for the treatment of bladder pain syndrome) can be used to attempt to recoat the bladder. After the medication recently underwent a great deal of scrutiny due to its possible causal relationship to retinopathy (harms the eyes), the FDA recently prompted a label update to include warnings, precautions, and information about adverse reactions. In addition to this known risk, this medication takes approximately six months to start working and can cause symptoms such as hair loss and GI-distress, making it difficult for many to stay compliant.

What's the cocktail, Doc?

Here's the thing. Every practitioner has a different cocktail. Most will include a combination of the following:

- **Anesthetic (such as lidocaine or bupivacaine):** The rationale is that anesthetics hold anti-inflammatory properties and also can be used as a strategy for diagnosis and therapy. Think of it this way: If we add a numbing agent to the cocktail and a patient exhibits symptomatic relief, then theoretically some of their pain must be coming from their bladder. In the field this is known as an anesthetic challenge, and it is key in the diagnosis and management of IC/BPS.
- **Coating agent:** Such agents include heparin or pentosan polysulfate. I know what you might be thinking: Heparin is a blood thinner, isn't it? Yes, when injected into the body, heparin is a blood thinner. However, when placed in the bladder it acts as an effective coating agent to help recoat that bladder.

- **Anti-inflammatory and steroid:** Considering that the concept of chronic inflammation and mast cell degranulation is the proposed pathophysiology behind IC/BPS, then decreasing inflammation by way of a localized steroid into the bladder is thought to be helpful. As of this writing, there are thought to be no systemic side effects of administration in this particular way.

- **Antibiotic:** Some gurus in the field will argue to place an antibiotic such as gentamicin in instillations, as we are learning more and more about the bladder microbiome and its effects and discrepancies in patients with IC/BPS. There is currently no right or wrong answer, simply personal preference based on practitioner and patient.

- **DMSO:** Also known as dimethyl sulfoxide, this substance can and does make you smell like garlic. It also can make symptoms worse before they get better, and for that reason is generally used as a last resort. This medication can also cause retinopathy, and patients who use it regularly require frequent ophthalmologic evaluations.

Do I get instillations forever?

Everyone does this differently because there are no set protocols or guidelines. But in my opinion, the answer is no. While utilizing bladder coating agents via instillations is thought to address the main pathophysiological process at the root of IC/BPS symptoms, we must remember that the remodeling of pathways takes time. This explains why most treatments show a gradually increasing benefit with longer treatment courses.

Many will recommend weekly or biweekly instillations for six to eight weeks in an effort to properly recoat the bladder. Some will recommend self-teaching for at-home instillations. Others will add substances such as sodium bicarbonate to increase penetration into the bladder wall, which in turn allows patients to taper off treatments and ultimately to use instillations as needed. No two courses are exactly the same, but understanding instillations, how and when they are used, and their benefits is important.

Some patients will feel like they have difficulty emptying their bladder after the procedure due to the lidocaine. For others this same treatment will provide a needed reprieve from the persistent urgency and frequency that plagues their everyday quality of life. Weekly catheterizations when done by sterile method are not thought to increase the number of urinary tract infections—this has been proven by the data. But for some, the simple act of catheterizing can create a profound refractory urethral pain.

So what's the lowdown on instillations? Ultimately, it varies on an individual basis. For some, this is an extremely beneficial form of treatment. For others, it is used just to break the cycle. Know your options, understand why they may or may not work, and properly discuss all the risks and benefits for your individual case with your treating doctor.

INJECTIONS

You're going to put that needle where?
Injections in the form of nerve blocks, trigger points, or neurotoxins (namely, Botox—don't let that word scare you) are currently pretty standard of care in the pelvic pain world for things like pudendal

neuralgia, neuropathic upregulation or neuroproliferation, and pelvic floor dysfunction. There are many different directions you can go when discussing injections. It is important to understand the risks and benefits of each, and then to utilize them appropriately for pain relief. Understanding the science behind injections, even in the form of dry needling (such as with acupuncture), can help provide you with a stepping-stone path for individualized care.

First off, what is a trigger point? And can it really occur in the pelvis? I get these questions a ton. And I think a basic understanding of the science behind trigger points is important because it gives you the power to understand which certain behaviors you may knowingly or unknowingly be doing that can be exacerbating your pelvic pain.

Myofascial trigger points are tender "knots" in taut muscle bands that produce pain. The pain, which may be local or referred, can produce a twitch response, or quiver, when these areas are touched. Furthermore, the pain associated with trigger points may be attributed to high local concentrations of inflammatory mediators, neuropeptides, and neurotransmitters. In a word: inflammation!

Diagnosing and understanding the science behind these areas helps to direct therapy via medication, physical therapy, trigger point injections, or Botox. Although the use of injectable agents to treat pelvic pain has not been well studied as of this writing, many experts in the field of pelvic pain include this tool as adjunctive therapy.

Trigger points differ from tender points but are a key aspect in the diagnosis and treatment of pelvic floor dysfunction. With trigger point injections we take a long spinal needle (not as scary as it looks but transparency is key, right?) and actually needle these areas of muscle that are causing pain and spasm.

Some of the data on injections and needling stem from acupuncture data. There are multiple studies that look at trigger point injections. My advice: Do your research to know the data!

Trigger Point Injections

Trigger point injections have been found to be effective in conjunction with physical therapy to treat pelvic pain. It's important to note this caveat: Injecting a muscle without utilizing physical therapy won't lead to long-term results. Part of the healing process involves needling or injecting these areas while simultaneously retraining the muscles with physical therapy. Needling without having a specialist help release the muscle isn't considered standard of care.

Studies have shown that dry needling is just as effective as trigger point injections, which can utilize anesthetic medications such as lidocaine and bupivacaine. So why use these anesthetics? Because we believe these medications also harbor anti-inflammatory properties that can be very helpful to hypertonic pelvic floors. As with any procedure, it's most successful when performed on the right patient in the right setting. The only way to do this is to know the data, respect the data, and to follow evidence-based guidelines.

Botox

Botox has demonstrated effectiveness in the treatment of several pain disorders, including focal dystonia, temporomandibular disorder, refractory myofascial pain syndrome, and tension- and migraine-type headaches. These positive results of using Botox to manage pain stimulated interest in its use for treating genitourinary pain conditions.

Botox's mechanism of action for pain relief is thought to be primarily based on the elimination of tonic muscle contraction and, subsequently, blunting nociceptive responses. Botox acts in decreasing the presynaptic release of acetylcholine at the neuromuscular junction. This is what causes the "paralysis" that Botox is known for (although it's somewhat of a misnomer or "bad rap" in my opinion). In addition, Botox has been shown to inhibit central glutamate, thus diminishing excitatory amino acid receptors that are important to the central windup process and pain perception.

Although adverse effects of botulinum toxin A are extremely rare, they have been reported. Botox is not a permanent treatment and positive results vary, lasting from 3 months to up to 12 months in some cases. Adverse effects are self-limiting and typically resolve as the medication begins to lose its potency. Patients must be fully informed and give their consent to all possible adverse effects and reactions prior to injections.

When used correctly, Botox is helpful in treating hypertonic pelvic floor dysfunction and certain types of vulvodynia. I like Botox (when used correctly) because of its longevity. It allows time for the body to reset. As with Botox use anywhere in the body, it is my opinion that less is more. Doses can range anywhere from 20 units to 300 units, although the higher the dosage the bigger the risk of side effects.

The risks of injecting Botox to the pelvic floor include bleeding, infection, urinary retention, or fecal incontinence. However, Botox to the pelvic floor is thought to be pretty safe (and I can confirm this from personal experience), as side effects as demonstrated in research occurred only in dosages of 200 units and above.

Less is more. An optimal benefit of neuromuscular release without the documented side effects can often be reached by simply using less of this medication. Based on my patients' experience, I've found that Botox often provides a great deal of benefit for those suffering from certain types of pelvic pain. We just need to wait to see what the FDA does in terms of assessing whether utilization for treating pelvic pain can be considered "on-label" (or approved for use for the diagnosis of pelvic floor dysfunction).

Nerve Blocks

Nerves play a pivotal role in pelvic pain disorders. And nerve blocks, and in certain cases bathing the nerves with anesthetics and anti-inflammatories, can be helpful for symptom relief. Nerve blocks involve injecting an anesthetic near a specific nerve or bundle of nerves to block sensations of pain arising from that specific area of the body. The obvious issue is longevity because nerve blocks typically don't last longer than the half-life of the local anesthesia. Nerve blocks provide an excellent diagnostic and therapeutic tool, kind of like a road map, to determine which nerves may be "revved up" in certain processes.

Important nerves in pelvic pain are:

- Ilioinguinal nerve
- Iliohypogastric nerve
- Genitofemoral nerve
- Pudendal nerve
- Lumbar plexus
- Superior hypogastric plexus
- Ganglion impar

One of the biggest factors to successfully implementing nerve blocks in the treatment of pelvic pain disorders is the importance of a multidisciplinary team. Nerve blocks can be excellent adjunctive therapies to other more long-term options such as Botox, and by virtue provide excellent diagnostic utility.

12

AT HOME

YOU ARE WHAT YOU EAT!
As with any change to your nutritional plan, you should take into account any dietary restrictions, food allergies or sensitivities, and any other special dietary needs that you may have. I hope that the information provided in this chapter will help you better understand any specific nutritional guidance your health care provider or nutritionist may give you as part of your tailored treated plan—if so, you should be sure to follow that guidance.

That there is a synergistic relationship between diet and well-being is beyond doubt. With the discovery that vitamins and minerals eradicate deficiency diseases, the role of these essential resources in maintaining health and mitigating disease has been confirmed, supporting the centuries-old concept of "food as medicine." This can be both positive and negative. Some foods and beverages can have harmful effects, such as increasing the risk of cardiovascular disease, inflammatory diseases, and even neoplastic disease (tumors). By controlling our intakes we can profoundly affect our quality of life. Understanding and implementing dietary modifications as an integral component of care is perhaps one of the most important—and easiest—things anyone can do for themselves.

When I walk through a grocery store and see fruits and vegetables, my mind immediately darts to their phytochemical properties. Unfortunately for some patients, foods act as triggers: triggers to their bladder pain, triggers to their yeast infections and vulvar pain, triggers to their bowels. In this chapter, we will examine these triggers in more detail.

I have always believed in taking a holistic approach to pelvic pain. That means looking at all factors—including health history, lifestyle, and diet choices—to create a customized treatment plan to help patients find relief. I've said it once, and I'll say it a million times over: The causes of pelvic pain are multifactorial. It's never as easy as saying your pain was caused by this or that. In almost all cases of pelvic pain there are many contributing factors at work.

As we continue to learn more about the nuances of pelvic pain, there's increasing support for the theory that diet could have a significant impact on pelvic pain symptoms. Inflammation is a known cause of chronic pain, and it's well documented that inflammation is often caused by the foods we eat. Additionally, pelvic pain conditions such as endometriosis, interstitial cystitis, and irritable bowel syndrome are all characterized by chronic inflammation. As the body of evidence grows, we can't ignore the role of diet in pelvic pain.

I encourage you to read this chapter through, and then read it over again. One of the biggest pitfalls of modern medicine is its ability to "fix" symptoms without addressing prevention and triggers. Don't get caught in that trap.

THE BENEFITS OF NUTRITION

Eat the rainbow!

You probably hear that phrase all the time. But there's truth in it. For many with bladder and pelvic pain, certain colorful foods can be triggers. We'll get to that in a bit. But first, let's discuss the nutrients and medicinal properties of certain foods based on color.

Red: Think tomatoes, bell peppers, and carrots. These foods contain lycopene, which is a carotenoid (a plant pigment with protective health benefits). It is believed that lycopene is protective against heart disease and genetic damage that can contribute to certain cancers.

Blue-Purple: Think eggplants, beets, red cabbage, and purple potatoes. These foods contain anthocyanins, which help prevent blood clots, delay cell aging, and may even help slow the onset of Alzheimer's disease.

Green: Think broccoli, Brussels sprouts, bok choy, cabbage, cauliflower, kale, collards, and arugula. These foods contain phytochemicals, bioflavonoids such as sulforaphane, isocyanates, and indoles, which inhibit carcinogens and boost detoxification. (Spa day for the gut!)

Pale and White (sometimes with a hint of green): Think garlic, onions, leeks, and other vegetables that contain allicins, which have powerful anticancer, antitumor, immune-boosting, and antimicrobial properties. These vegetables also contain antioxidant flavonoids like quercetin and kaempferol.

Orange: Think carrots, pumpkin, acorn and winter squash, and sweet potatoes. They contain alpha-carotene, which protects against cancer and benefits both eyesight and skin changes.

Yellow and Green: Think spinach; collard, mustard, and turnip greens; yellow corn; peas; and avocado. (This is a tricky category, because they don't always appear yellow to the eye.) These foods contain lutein and zeaxanthin, which help eye health and the treatment of atherosclerosis.

THE LINK BETWEEN DIET AND PELVIC PAIN

Chronic inflammation from pelvic pain conditions can severely compromise your quality of life. Painful periods, pain during urination and bowel movements, painful sex, gastrointestinal issues . . . these symptoms cannot be ignored. Many theories exist for how chronic inflammation develops—including genetic, hormonal, structural, and autoimmune causes—but often no true cause can be identified.

This is where diet may come into the picture. Certain foods are believed to increase inflammation in the body and, as a result, may aggravate pelvic pain. For example, the pain associated with endometriosis is largely caused by inflammation in the uterus and surrounding organs. Because of this, experts recommend a diet rich in anti-inflammatory foods, such as fruits and vegetables, omega-3 fats, whole grains, beans, and legumes. Inflammation-causing foods, such as red meats, processed foods, alcohol, and caffeine, have been linked to an increase in endometriosis symptoms, so it's best to reduce (or remove) these things from your diet. While some foods may exacerbate your pain, others may help reduce your symptoms. Changing your diet could help you find relief. Here are some ideas to get you started:

1. Up Your Omega-3 Intake

Omega-3s are healthy, anti-inflammatory fats found in fish and many plant-based sources. They're known to relieve pain and are believed to counteract the inflammation brought on by conditions such as endometriosis. Aim to have three to five servings of high-fat fish per week, two to four servings of cold-pressed vegetable oil per day, or start taking an omega-3 supplement. Increasing your daily intake of omega-3 fats is one of the simplest changes you can make to your diet.

Best sources: wild salmon, herring, sardines, black cod; extra virgin olive oil, flaxseed oil, nut-based oils.

2. Load Up on Fruits and Veggies

It should come as no surprise that fruits and vegetables are major players in any healthy diet. Not only are fruits and veggies anti-inflammatory and chock-full of antioxidants, they're also full of fiber, which promotes healthy digestion and may help to lower estrogen levels. Fruits and veggies also provide plenty of essential nutrients that work to reduce pain in the body. Try to eat four to five servings of fruits and vegetables every day. Choose organic whenever possible and eat the rainbow of colors to get a wide variety of vitamins and minerals.

But be careful: Certain fruits and vegetables (specifically those acidic in nature, such as lemons, limes, oranges, and spicy peppers) can often exacerbate bladder and pelvic floor–based symptoms. As noted at the beginning of this chapter, it's important to address dietary issues with your physician so together you can come up with an individualized dietary plan that suits your specific conditions. The list of foods noted here is in no way comprehensive, given how individualized dietary triggers may be.

Best sources: dark, leafy greens (spinach, kale, collard greens), cruciferous veggies (cauliflower, broccoli, Brussels sprouts), beets, berries, stone fruits (peaches, nectarines, plums), apples, pears, and more.

3. Reduce Trans Fats

As much as omega-3 fats can work wonders on inflammation, trans fats do the exact opposite. Found in many processed foods, trans fats have been linked to heart disease, increased inflammation in the body, and in some studies, an increased incidence of pelvic pain conditions. Avoiding these foods could help to reduce your symptoms.

Foods to avoid: processed foods like crackers, cookies, pastries, and more.

4. Cut Down on Red Meat

Red meats are linked to hormonal imbalances and are known to increase inflammation in the body, both of which may contribute to an increase in pelvic pain symptoms. Aim to reduce your intake to a maximum of one to two servings per week, and I recommend that you choose organic or grass-fed meats when possible.

Foods to reduce: beef, pork, veal.

5. Eat Your Beans (and Legumes)

Beans are good for more than your heart—they're full of folic acid, magnesium, potassium, and soluble fiber. Magnesium in particular is known to have anti-inflammatory properties and fiber, as we've mentioned; it also may lower estrogen levels, which can reduce symptoms of endometriosis. Legumes and beans are also low glycemic, meaning they help to stabilize blood sugars, which can reduce inflammation.

Best sources: lentils, chickpeas, black beans.

6. Increase Whole Grains

Whole grains are known to balance blood sugar, reducing spikes that cause inflammation. They also provide important B vitamins and fiber, which promote healthy digestion and decrease inflammation in the gut. While a totally gluten-free diet is not necessary unless you have celiac disease, gluten sensitivity, a wheat allergy, or another such condition, reducing gluten may help to calm pain from certain pelvic pain conditions. Aim for two to four servings of whole grains a day. This may seem like a lot, but servings of whole grains are "ounce equivalent," meaning that the portion size equals the amount of food that weighs one ounce. Examples of ounce equivalents include one slice of bread; a half cup of cooked oatmeal, pasta, or rice; an ounce of crackers; or a cup of dry cold cereal.

Best sources: brown rice, quinoa, buckwheat, steel-cut oats.

More research is required to fully understand the link between diet and pelvic pain. But until we know more, my view is that making conscious changes to your diet is a simple way to take one aspect of your holistic treatment into your own hands. If nothing else, you should benefit from a healthier lifestyle. And that will take you one step closer to living a healthier life.

ELIMINATION DIET

Some foods can actually trigger and increase bladder discomfort in certain individuals.

The concept of dietary triggers and bladder pain may be related to what's known as leaky gut. If you have a potential degradation in the protective GAG layer of the bladder, and you consume certain foods that are irritative to the bladder, then you are more likely to trigger painful sensations. That is, you will have tripped what we call a dietary trigger.

In order to figure out which foods you should avoid, you might want to try an elimination diet (subject, of course, to your health care provider's input). Although elimination diets can be good to practice over short periods of time to isolate intolerances and sensitivities to certain foods, over the long term their restrictive nature can result in severe nutrient deficiencies and malnutrition, which can negatively impact the microbiome.

How to Begin

Before we get into the nitty-gritty of starting an elimination diet, I'm here to tell you that not *all* acidic or spicy foods are triggers for everyone. Yes. Read that again. All too many times in my practice I've seen patients restrict foods that may *not* be culprits so heavily that they become nutritionally deficient.

Some data suggest that almost 80 percent of patients with IC/BPS are diet-sensitive. Eighty percent! Is that right? No, it's wrong. Remember what I said about cherry-picking the data? Dietary studies tend to be heavily confounded due to high amounts of selection bias. More often than not they are questionnaire-based studies, and the people who tend to respond to the questionnaires tend to be . . . you guessed it . . . diet sensitive. That said, also take everything I say in this section with a "grain of salt." (See what I did there, a little diet humor for you.) I believe it is always important to discuss all treatment options with your physician or dietician as much of this involves an individualized spin.

The cardinal rule of starting elimination diets is to write down foods that you think may be triggers.

How do I know which foods are potential triggers?
Generally speaking, these are foods that increase *pain* anywhere in your body within 15 minutes to 6 hours after you ingest them.

This can be pain with the bladder as it fills, urethral pain, or burning vaginal pain. Remember to distinguish between pain and frequency. Many things like alcohol and caffeine can increase urinary frequency, but these are not necessarily considered triggers, as the mechanism by which they increase frequency can occur in people with or without pelvic pain syndromes.

So if I think a food may be a dietary trigger, what is the best way to proceed?

A two-week to one-month washout period, eating only pelvic-friendly foods, should be started in order to properly control and to test the hypothesis of bothersome foods. (In my practice, I have found that one month is too long for many patients to remain compliant.) After the washout period, a methodical reintroduction of a suspected trigger food should be done so as to monitor its effect on symptoms.

Day 1: Small (partial) portion.
Day 2: If no symptoms appear, consume a slightly larger amount.
Day 3: If no flaring continues, test a regular-size portion.

Clinical experience suggests a three-day waiting period between the introduction of each test food. Do not add any challenge (meaning trigger) foods back into the regular daily diet until completing this testing protocol for all foods. The use of a food diary is a very effective tool to help you enhance the awareness of your food intake. I think it's a very valuable contributor to the success of a testing plan.

Diets tend to embrace fads. We can spend hours discussing diets like low oxalate, FODMAP, and gluten-free, but the data in relation to pelvic pain disorders is variable. In addition, the data regarding diets and pelvic pain is very skewed, ultimately creating restrictive patterns that can result in nutritional depletion.

My advice: Take your time, understand your triggers (if they exist), but don't restrict yourself simply based on, say, something you read on the internet. Understand that the recent increase in interest in this topic has unfortunately also caused the spread of a great deal of misinformation. The touting of generalizations has led people to eliminate more foods and beverages than necessary. In an effort to alleviate pain, people often abstain from healthy foods, possibly leading to nutritional deficiencies. Limiting nutrients can be damaging and counterproductive to patients who need to fortify their immunity, nerve transmission, wound healing, blood flow, and overall health. Weigh your options and proceed with caution by understanding the facts behind diet and pain!

PHYTOTHERAPY

Pelvic pain adversely affects the life of many patients, and the management of this pain can prove frustrating and dissatisfying to both patient and practitioner. While the body of literature regarding pelvic pain is growing, the evidence surrounding conventional medical therapies is controversial. With so many unmet needs and continued questions, many people are turning to alternative supplements. In particular, interest in phytotherapy (using plant-derived products as medical therapy) has increased. Such therapies have been popular in other countries, but their use in the United States has only recently started to increase.

There are many "plus points" when introducing alternative treatments. Phytotherapy, for example, does have several potential advantages such as low cost, fewer side effects compared to many prescription medications, and unique mechanisms of action. One difficulty with utilizing phytotherapy in practice is the lack of standardization of these products, because there are wide variations depending on brand or dose. Unlike pharmaceuticals, phytotherapy products are not regulated by the Food and Drug Administration (FDA). As such, companies selling these products are not required to prove efficacy, safety, or even the actual presence of the advertised active ingredient. If you decide to try phytotherapy, it is important that you understand the phytochemicals involved so as to ensure that you are not purchasing products that are worthless, or even worse, harmful.

SUPPLEMENTS

One of my biggest qualms with medicine is its focus on interventional strategies by way of medications and procedures, without adequately addressing prevention strategies. Any unifying theory of modern medicine, insofar as one exists, will need to incorporate nontraditional treatment modalities to complement traditional ones. If traditional medications are not providing adequate relief from your symptoms, there are certain dietary supplements that have shown promise in the treatment of pelvic pain. While supplements are important, there's not enough good data around efficacy. I find that a lot of patients benefit from supplements, but only at the right dosage. Not overdoing it is important, as there is a certain point where supplements can also be harmful. However, supplements, in my opinion, can be an important tool for prevention and can decrease the frequency and severity of relapses or flares.

Quercetin

This antioxidant fights inflammation, and it may be effective in treating nonbacterial prostatitis.

What is quercetin?
It is a bioflavonoid, meaning that it's a substance that naturally occurs and can be found in many foods and consumables. For example, quercetin is found in red wine, green tea, onions, and garlic. Citrus foods, apples, parsley, and sage also contain this powerful antioxidant.

How does quercetin work?
Quercetin inhibits production of inflammatory cytokines, specifically IL-6, IL-8, and TNF.

What does this mean?
It stops the production of compounds within our bodies that lead to increases in inflammation. Interestingly, this is one of the only supplements that has empirical data (in the form of double-blind placebo controlled trials) to demonstrate its efficacy. In one study using pain scores, 82 percent of patients receiving the medication showed at least 25 percent improvement. This is quite substantial.

Overall, in my experience, quercetin therapy is very well tolerated. Some common side effects include nausea, joint pain, and for men, orange pigmentation to the semen.

D-Mannose

This is an anti-inflammatory sugar that can provide relief for those experiencing recurrent urinary tract infections (UTIs) and interstitial cystitis (IC).

What is D-mannose?
D-mannose is a naturally occurring sugar found in some plants and fruits (cranberry and pineapple, for example).

How does D-mannose work?
Research has shown that D-mannose may provide urinary tract support by inhibiting the attachment of E. coli bacteria to the urinary tract and thereby helping to prevent infection. In certain studies, 2 grams of D-mannose daily was effective in preventing UTIs, with only 15 percent of women with recurring UTIs getting another one after starting the supplement (as compared to 60 percent who didn't take anything).

Common side effects can include diarrhea and nausea.

Aloe Vera

Aloe vera can also improve symptoms of interstitial cystitis (IC), with some studies reporting 63 to 68 percent improvement in pelvic pain.

Concentrated aloe vera has been used by thousands of patients to reduce the symptoms of interstitial cystitis. Although the mechanism of action of aloe vera has not been proven, it is hypothesized that the ability of aloe vera to increase the body's production of glycosaminoglycan (GAG) molecules—which has been demonstrated in the healing of wounds—may also increase GAG synthesis in the bladder lining, where the GAG layer plays an important role in shielding the tissue of the bladder from irritants in the urine. Orally administered aloe vera has been demonstrated in preclinical studies to increase the body's synthesis of GAG molecules by 43 percent. It has also shown the ability to increase both types of GAG molecules—both sulfated and nonsulfated molecules—which form the bladder lining's protective layer. In a pilot randomized, double-blind clinical trial, oral treatment with aloe vera was able to reduce IC symptoms in nearly 90 percent of patients over a three-month treatment course. These results were confirmed in a survey of more than 400 IC patients. After three months of treatment, 75 percent of patients surveyed noted relief from at least one IC symptom, while nearly half reported significant relief from the majority of their symptoms.

Vitamin D

Vitamin D, believe it or not, is an important supplement both for urinary and vaginal health. It is involved in the production of antimicrobial peptides, substances that fight off infection-causing bacteria, fungi, and viruses as these pathogens try to move into organs and through mucous membranes. Researchers have recently found evidence supporting that higher vitamin D levels offer especially strong protection against urinary tract infections (UTIs). Vitamin D may be a potential complement in the prevention of UTI. This is especially important as the advent of multidrug-resistant bacteria have become more common. There is a question as to whether determining the vitamin D status of individuals with a history of UTI may be of importance in terms of evaluating their ability to fend off intruding bacteria.

Here's why: Anatomically, the urinary tract is frequently exposed to infection-causing agents and therefore has a built-in, rapid-defense system led by the antimicrobial peptide known as cathelicidin. When pathogens threaten, cathelicidin is secreted by bladder epithelial cells. Interestingly, vitamin D actually increases the expression of this peptide. This is particularly notable when the bladder cells were infected with E. coli (one of the most common causes of UTIs). Studies have observed a significant increase in cathelicidin expression when E. coli is present in those who took vitamin D_3 supplementation. This is beneficial because the overuse of antibiotics, aside from increasing resistance patterns, can also wreak havoc on the "good" bacteria that are often protective (the microbiome). Therefore, if in fact vitamin D produces only this germ-killing peptide in the presence of harmful bacteria such as E. coli, there should be a theoretic protective effect on the microbiome, leaving the "good" bacteria potentially unharmed. These findings are totally neat and new, but the prospect of this work and the potential benefit of this supplement is astounding.

Constipation Supplements

Being constipated nearly always causes pain, and it can make existing pelvic pain worse. It can increase symptoms in both the pelvic floor and bladder, influencing frequency and urgency, and it often interferes with issues of sitting and movement. There are a plethora of mechanisms by which this occurs, including the concept of pelvic organ cross talk (or viscerovisceral convergence) known as the bowel-bladder connection. But this also occurs by way of simple, anatomical pathophysiology. Constipation leads to an increase in the hypertonicity of pelvic floor musculature, while pelvic floor hypertonicity can lead to increased constipation. There are several supplements that can help with this, including:

Flaxseed oil: Flaxseed oil may help to reduce gastrointestinal symptoms and to relieve constipation. The benefits are that it is gentle and does not increase contractions of the GI tract, which can often lead to diarrhea and pain.

Magnesium: Taking magnesium supplements can help to provide relief from constipation. However, magnesium has a secondary benefit of supporting muscle and nerve function, especially in those with pelvic floor dysfunction. A double benefit!

Epsom salts: Warm baths with Epsom salts have been shown to relieve constipation. Heat in and of itself helps to relax muscles, thereby increasing capillary blood flow to the area, which helps to keep muscles relaxed.

Probiotics

While we will delve into the nitty-gritty of probiotics in Chapter 13, I think it's important to touch on probiotics when discussing supplements. Probiotics can be a frustrating subject for both the patient and doctor because the data on probiotics is conflicting. While the claims on many specific probiotics and their utility have been called into question, there are a few strains that the data support for pelvic health. Let's quickly go over them.

Lactobacillus (L. reuteri): This important strain is helpful in balancing the pH of the vagina, with theoretic benefit against recurrent yeast and bacterial vaginosis.

Lactobacillus (L. rhamnosus): This strain has been shown to have anti-inflammatory benefits and to improve gut mucosal barrier function ("leaky gut syndrome"), as well as to reduce anxiety.

Saccharomyces (S. boulardii): This strain can help lower inflammation, which is promising with patients who experience symptoms of bowel-bladder or viscerovisceral convergence.

Bifidobacterium (B. breve): This strain has been shown to ease digestion, boost immunity, and play an important role in immune function and allergy response. It also can help with compromised gut mucosal barrier function and may reduce anxiety, too.

Zinc

Zinc can be an important supplement in men (or penis owners). There are several studies that have validated the efficacy of zinc in the management of prostatitis, specifically category IIIB CP/CPPS (chronic prostatitis/chronic pelvic pain syndrome). The therapeutic dose tends to be anywhere over 200 mg (as with other supplements, it is important not to overdo the dosing recommendations). Studies found that men taking approximately 200 to 220 mg of zinc experienced a decrease both in pain and voiding symptoms such as frequency, urgency, and difficulty starting a stream. This data may also be helpful for those who suffer from pelvic floor dysfunction, as the causes for inflammation and discrete trigger and tender points seems to be analogous with these disorders. In addition, microbial studies of the prostate glands revealed that zinc was helpful in inhibiting bacterial growth.

Side effects, which are especially found with excessive zinc consumption (200 to 300 mg), include nausea, vomiting, muscle cramps, diarrhea, lethargy, and visual changes, including color blindness. Again, although supplements are seemingly innocuous, overconsumption of them can lead to harmful side effects, although reportedly usually temporary in nature.

WE ARE ALL CONNECTED

While we tend to look at our bodies as separate systems and approach care in a problem-based fashion, in doing so we lose sight of understanding the human body as a whole. My philosophy is always patient-centered not problem-centered care.

The abdominopelvic cavity is the largest hollow space in the body. It is bounded at the top by the diaphragm muscles, which separate it from the chest cavity, and is bounded at the bottom by the pelvic floor muscles. Inside the cavity are the body's urinary, digestive, and reproductive organs—critical for life's most vital functions. Protecting and supporting those organs is an array of other muscles, nerves, tissues, fascia, and linking ligaments that hold everything together. While I am painting a simplistic picture here, I want you to be aware of how our bodies function as a whole, both anatomically and physiologically.

Our bodies' natural response to pain is to protect, often via clenching maneuvers. An example is when you clench your jaw when you're in pain or stressed. This is an important aspect of how our bodies function, because over time the muscle tightening, squeezing, and clenching can lead to muscles locking into a short, tight, and painful state. In the medical world, we call this hyperto-nicity. This is a problem because when those muscles and fascia become "locked" together, they become less flexible, less effective in their job of controlling movement—enhancing stability and ulti-mately protecting the organs within the core of the body.

Because the muscles of the pelvic floor are attached to the skel-eton, their response to pain extends beyond the pelvis region. How so? If you contract your pelvic floor muscles, they in turn will pull on your tailbone, your pubic bone, your lower back, and your hip bone. By doing so, your skeletal alignment is altered. Imagine what might happen if the muscles in the pelvic floor experience hyper-tonicity. Could your backache, butt pain, and pain down the leg be related to problems in your pelvic floor? Absolutely.

This is how "the tug of war" begins. Let's think about it this way: Our natural state as humans is to stand upright—vertical against gravity. If a muscle shortens or tightens or begins to tug your body over to a particular side, it's only reflexive that another part of our musculature will try to pull the body back the other way to maintain that vertical alignment. In this regard, you can think of the body as a "pulley-lever" system that seeks balance. Makes sense? Let's call this the "muscle tug of war." As this tug of war continues, some muscles work overtime, leading to continued hypertonicity, tight-ening, taut or tender bands, and pain.

Now let's take this a step further and break some myths.

Somehow, there appears to be this notion that tight muscles are strong muscles. In fact, the opposite is true. Think of a bicep: If you have tight and even painful muscles in your arm from overworking it, can you lift less or more? You guessed it—less! Tight muscles are, in fact, weak muscles. Now, what connects muscle to muscle or ligaments? Connective tissue. When this tissue becomes restricted (due to the tightening and hypertonicity of surrounding muscles), capillary blood flow decreases. This means that the blood that we need to nourish these nerves, muscles, and tissues, and to remove waste, decreases. In the pelvic area specifically, this can lead to changes in the epithelium or mucosa in various areas, which is often exemplified by thinning of the skin, architectural changes of the vaginal mucosa, and alteration of the pH balance. For example, have you ever gotten that "pins and needles" sensation when your leg falls asleep? It's a result of changes in capillary blood flow and downstream neuromuscular changes. This is important to note, as most who experience burning or pain tend to attribute these symptoms to infection or inflammation, when often the culprit is neuromuscular and blood flow changes.

Let's keep going. When neuromuscular and blood flow changes occur, it affects joints and urinary, reproductive, and gastrointestinal organs. These changes are often accompanied by an uptick in inflammation (which itself may be a root cause) and can absolutely affect appropriate functioning of your entire body.

We are all connected.

Common symptoms of pelvic floor dysfunction are often described with phrases such as:

- "I feel like I have a golf ball stuck in my vagina."
- "It feels like a feather tickling my bladder."
- "I feel a great deal of pressure that worsens with sitting for long periods of time."
- "Constipation always makes me feel worse, in fact it increases my frequency and urgency."
- "It's hard for me to start a stream and I feel like I don't empty."
- "Wearing tight clothes increases my discomfort."

Muscles in your pelvic floor are just like muscles in other areas of your body in that they have "muscle memory." Long periods of time in a taut state brings to light the importance of muscle retraining, often in the form of physical therapy. Making sure your physical body is aligned and tension-free is an important integrative step that can complement medications, procedures, and interventions. And that is best accomplished by first understanding the interconnectedness of the body as a whole.

PELVIC PHYSICAL THERAPY AND TOOLS FOR SELF-TREATMENT

Many health care providers recommend pelvic floor physical therapy as either a primary or adjunctive intervention for treating pelvic pain. And I agree! Pelvic floor physical therapy is one of the most important aspects in understanding how our bodies respond to pain and what we can do intrinsically to help ourselves.

Pelvic physical therapy is a highly specialized form of rehabilitation conducted by a physical therapist (PT) who has undergone training in examination and treatment of pelvic floor dysfunction. Pelvic floor physical therapy addresses various issues of the pelvic floor muscles (PFM), hips, lower back, and abdomen. As noted elsewhere in this book, the pelvic floor is a group of muscles, tendons, ligaments, and fascia that form a sling-like hammock from the pubic bone to the tailbone and laterally to the bony protuberances that you sit on. They support the abdominal and pelvic organs (the bladder, uterus, and rectum) and assist in maintaining upright posture. These muscles are important for maintaining control of the bladder and bowel and in sexual activity. Pelvic floor muscle dysfunction (PFMD) includes a variety of issues that occur when the muscles of the pelvic floor are not functioning properly.

The PFM can become underactive, weak, or lose coordination after pregnancy, delivery, or surgery. The muscles can also be injured with repetitive straining, such as with chronic constipation, repetitive heavy lifting, and some impact sports. When the pelvic floor muscles become weakened, urinary incontinence, fecal incontinence, and pelvic organ prolapse (POP) can occur. Specifically, when the muscles and ligaments supporting a woman's pelvic organs weaken, the organs within the pelvis (including the bladder, uterus, and rectum) can drop lower in the pelvis, creating a bulge in the vagina—this is known as prolapse.

On the other hand, the PFM can become overactive, or too tight, which can contribute to general pelvic pain, constipation, and issues with penetrative sex. Often trigger points or tender points develop in the PFM that can further contribute to pain and loss of function. These are similar to the "knots" that you might find in your neck or back, that when you press on them, they are tender, and when you massage them, it relieves the pain.

Due to the complex nature of the anatomy and musculoskeletal functioning in this area, a detailed medical history, thorough examination, and unique plan of care needs to be developed by a pelvic physical therapist to treat the underlying issues. This care is delivered in conjunction with other treatments, including a team approach with primary care physicians, urologists, nurse practitioners, obstetrician-gynecologists (OB-GYN), gastroenterologists, oncologists, and other health care workers.

Pelvic physical therapists evaluate and treat a wide variety of pelvic floor and abdominal conditions in men, women, and transgender people. The conditions specific to women include but are not limited to:

- Bladder disorders
- Urinary incontinence
- Urinary urgency, frequency, hesitancy
- IC (interstitial cystitis)
- Bladder pain syndrome

- Bowel disorders
- IBS (irritable bowel syndrome)
- Constipation/incomplete emptying
- Pelvic pain conditions
- Levator ani syndrome (pressure or ache in the sacrum, coccyx, rectum, and vagina caused by overactivity of the levator ani muscles)
- Dyspareunia (pain with intercourse)
- Anorgasmia (difficulty achieving orgasm)
- Pudendal neuralgia
- Vulvodynia
- Vulvar vestibulitis
- Vaginismus
- Pelvic congestion
- Lichens sclerosis and lichens planus (skin conditions associated with pelvic pain)
- Coccydynia (pain in the tailbone region)
- Postsurgical conditions
- Hysterectomy
- Hernia
- Laparoscopy, including endometriosis excision
- Caesarean section
- Appendectomy
- Post-cancer treatments
- Lymphedema
- Post-radiation pelvic pain

What Does the First Visit of Pelvic Physical Therapy Look Like?

Based on the approach of the pelvic physical therapists who I work with, here's what you can expect: the first session of pelvic physical therapy is an initial evaluation. You will be asked to fill out forms to provide your pelvic physical therapist (PT) with your complete medical history that includes your current medications and other pertinent medical information. This visit will take place in a private room, and you are welcome to bring a partner, friend, or other chaperone for comfort. The pelvic PT will discuss your medical history and ask specific follow-up questions pertaining to how your bladder, bowels, and sexual organs have been functioning. This helps the therapist better understand what the driving factors of your condition are. A pelvic PT will seek to help you solve the underlying issue, not just treat the symptoms.

A physical examination will be performed. This includes an assessment of your posture, coordination, and an evaluation of your spine, hips, and often the knees and feet, as they can be associated with issues in the pelvis.

An external and intravaginal assessment of the pelvic floor muscles can be performed on the first visit, although sometimes this is deferred to later sessions depending on the time frame, needs, and desires of the individual patient. The visual examination allows the pelvic PT to see the tone, integrity, and vascularization of the vulva and superficial pelvic floor muscles. This assessment gives important information to the pelvic PT as to the overall health of the vulva and pelvic floor muscles.

For the internal assessment of the pelvic floor muscles, the therapist uses a gloved hand and just one or two fingers to assess the strength, endurance, and coordination of the pelvic floor muscles. The physical therapist will ask you to perform various types of pelvic floor muscle contractions (also called Kegel exercises), as well as ask you to elongate the pelvic floor by bearing down. Additionally, the therapist will assess areas of pain or tenderness inside the pelvic floor via the vagina or rectum. In some cases, particularly in the case of tailbone pain, a therapist might recommend a rectal assessment of the muscles and joints.

The first session will allow the pelvic PT to create an overall plan of care unique to your needs. The length of treatment may span from a few weeks to a few months depending on what your issue is, and how long your symptoms have been present.

Treatments consist of many different modalities of care. Manual therapy involves soft tissue mobilization, relief of trigger points, joint mobilizations, and scar tissue massage to restore PFM length and function of the muscles of the pelvis and abdomen. Biofeedback is a tool that allows the therapist to help you to "retrain" your muscles for better coordination. A sensor may be placed on the outside or inside of the body that is connected to a device that gives real-time feedback as to how your muscles are performing. Ultrasound imaging may also be utilized to observe your organs and pelvic floor for training purposes and to give the therapist additional information. Exercises that are tailored to help restore muscle functioning are an integral part of pelvic floor rehabilitation. These exercises may consist of specific forms of stretching, stability exercises, pelvic floor exercises, and overall wellness exercises.

Additionally, lifestyle changes might be part of the rehabilitation process as recommended by the PT after the assessment. As you know, certain foods, beverages, and habits can contribute to bowel and bladder dysfunction. Bladder irritants are often recommended to be limited so as to allow the bladder to heal and reset. Smoking affects the bladder, vasculature, and nerves in the pelvis—in addition to its other, even better-documented health risks—so your health care provider and PT will most likely strongly recommend that you stop smoking. Certain dietary changes might be suggested, as well.

Exercises for Pelvic Floor Relaxation and Down Training

Before starting any new exercise plan, you should consult with a professional. Exercises for pelvic floor relaxation are no exception. Subject to your health care provider's specific guidance, stretches and body positioning with breathing are generally a helpful component of the healing process for pelvic pain. The pelvic floor muscles respond well to stretches for the hip and low back; the hip and low back also share connective tissue (fascia) and shared nerves. The following poses and stretches can be performed any time of day, and, subject to your health care provider's guidance, it is recommended that you find the ones that work best for your body. This may include all of them or just one or two that are highly effective for you. During your exercises it is important to remain mindful of your breathing and to focus your attention on ensuring that the pelvic floor muscles remain relaxed and unclenched.

Child's pose: In this exercise, maintain an easy breath into the sides of the ribs and allow the relaxation, dropping, or "letting go" in the pelvic floor. Start by kneeling on the floor with your toes together and your knees hip-width apart. Rest the palms on top of your thighs. On the exhale, lower your torso between your knees. Extend your arms alongside your torso with your palms facing downward. Remember to relax your shoulder toward to the ground. This exercise can be adapted using a pillow to achieve a different sensation and release of the pelvic floor. This adaptation involves using a pillow either behind the knees or in the front fold of the hips.

Cave squat: A deep squat stretch can be done by grasping a kitchen counter, chair, or even leaning into a corner of the room for support. Try to keep your feet flat on the ground and spaced slightly wider than your hips. Drop your hips downward and breathe into the sides of the rib cage. Envision the pelvic floor dropping and releasing.

Cat and cow flow: Begin on your hands and knees. You may need to place a towel under your knees or wrists to relieve pressure on the joints. Inhale and lift your head slightly upward, arching the back, and bringing the abdomen downward toward the floor. Then exhale and press your back up toward the ceiling, direct your head and tailbone to the floor, and round the spine. Then inhale and reverse back down into the starting position. Repeat 10 to 20 times.

Hip rotator stretch: This exercise stretches the hip muscle that connects to the pelvic floor in the pelvic bowl. Hip mobility is an important component of a healthy pelvic floor. Begin by lying on your back. Cross your right ankle over your left knee and then lift your left knee up toward your chest. Hold for 30 seconds and then switch to the other leg. Repeat three times on each leg.

Adductor stretch: The adductor muscles are a group of muscles on the inner thigh that attach to the bottom of the pelvic bones on the right and left sides of the pelvic bowl. These muscles are commonly tight in people who experience pelvic, vulva, or vaginal pain. To do the adductor stretch, from a standing position, lunge to the left by bending the left knee and keeping the right leg straight. Press your hips back as if you were sitting in a chair and do not allow your left knee to move forward beyond the left foot. Repeat the same steps with the right side—lunge to the right by bending the right knee and keeping the left leg straight. Press hips back as if you were sitting in a chair and do not allow your right knee to move forward beyond the right foot. Do a maximum of 12 reps for each side.

There are many ways to manage your pelvic pain in conjunction with pelvic physical therapy. Working one-on-one with a pelvic therapist will help you achieve your goals. Consistency in using tools and performing self-care routines that include exercises and mindful breathing are imperative in the healing process. During this process you will learn more about yourself, your body, and what works for you. This is a highly individualized experience and although results will not be apparent overnight, by showing up for yourself consistently over time you will get there, and it will be worth it.

LIFESTYLE MODIFICATIONS

Lifestyle is an important aspect of health. The first step in a patient's understanding of the importance of lifestyle begins with patient education. Setting realistic goals and expectations right from the outset of care is essential in the treatment of pelvic pain and maintaining excellent pelvic health. I always like to make it clear to my patients that understanding pain involves understanding its chronicity. Incorporating lifestyle modifications is an excellent, sustainable mode of prevention of repetitive flares. Believe it or not, our lifestyle choices, often driven by our behavioral patterns, account for at least half of the preventable habits that cause disease. What's my point? What we do every single day matters.

Sleep (Get Your Zzzzz)

According to the National Sleep Foundation, adults need 7 to 9 hours of sleep per night, although some people may be fine with 6 hours and some may need up to 10 hours. Sleeping less than 7 to 8 hours has been linked to an increase in heart disease and stroke. Sleep is a lifestyle element that affects our lives in many ways.

Fragmented sleep in mice has been shown to lead to obesity and insulin resistance, and harmful alterations in the gut microbiome. These mice had increased levels of more pathogenic microbes and decreased levels of more good microbes, which led to inflammation. There is no doubt that sleep deprivation can increase your fat stores, your inflammation levels, and your intestinal permeability. The data is still out on whether we can extrapolate this to the bladder. Regardless, the lack of sleep and its relationship to inflammation should be explanatory enough.

Remember that not all sleep is created equal. Things such as alcohol, technology screens, and foods can affect your sleep patterns and can cause a lack of sleep. Adequate, good, restorative sleep absolutely has a drastic impact on your health, and, yes, ladies and gentlemen this includes your pelvic health. Sleep hygiene is also quite important. It is important to understand that quality of sleep is the foundation for optimal health and wellness.

Some good bedtime habits for optimal sleep:

- Utilizing blue light blockers and night screen mode
- Keeping a cool temperature (66 to 72°F)
- Morning sun exposure
- Daily movement
- Avoid screens 2 to 3 hours prior to bed
- Avoid heavy meals and alcohol intake prior to bed
- Avoid naps greater than 15 to 13 minutes
- Utilize breathwork and meditation
- Develop a consistent sleep schedule
- Use the bed for rest and sleep only

Getting a good night's sleep can be a struggle for those who suffer from pelvic pain and floor disorders. They may experience nocturia, which is waking up at night to urinate. Even utilizing simple sleep-aid supplements such as melatonin, which is thought to have anti-inflammatory effects, can be helpful in those who are struggling to get good-quality sleep. Certain medications can have side effects, such as lethargy and drowsiness, and these medications can be taken at night to turn the side effect into a support for better nighttime sleep.

Exercise

It has been said that just 30 minutes of moderate exercise three to four times a week delivers extraordinary health benefits. Exercise can certainly help you start your day strong by jump-starting your metabolic engine and helping to balance your brain chemistry, blood sugar, and hormones. Data suggests that Americans live a generally sedentary lifestyle, and that 88 percent of our population does not get enough exercise. While this sounds like a large number, it is actually not as surprising as you may think.

So how does something as benign as movement provide such dramatic benefit?

Improves insulin sensitivity: Many studies have shown how exercise actually increases insulin sensitivity within the cells of our bodies, including the muscles. With improved insulin sensitivity, our bodies need less insulin, so less is produced. Less insulin enables a decrease in blood sugar and less fat storage. Improved insulin sensitivity is also linked to a decrease in inflammation, which is important to pelvic health.

Reduces stress: Exercise is paramount in reducing stress. Have you ever felt the need to get in a good workout on days that feel extremely chaotic? A good workout is a great stress reliever. And that is because exercise reduces cortisol—a stress hormone that is the culprit for inflammation, insulin resistance, and fat storage. Cortisol also increases inflammatory cytokines. For my patients, what's important is incorporating specific exercises that help them to lengthen muscles without placing strain on the system.

Helps your brain function: An "exercised brain" is a happy brain. I mean this. Exercise has been proven to improve memory, learning, and concentration. Vigorous exercise helps to stimulate certain neuropathic pathways that help with depression, insomnia, and mood stability. Through the formation of brain-derived neurotrophic factor (BDNF) there is stimulation of neuroplasticity and changes in the firing patterns of neurotransmitters that are beneficial to brain function.

Improves sexual function: Yes! I always say sexual health is a marker of our overall health. It cannot and should not be ignored. Exercise helps to increase sexual function by increasing circulation throughout the body, which is important for arousal and orgasm, in addition to increasing energy. One of the biggest hurdles in maintaining a healthy sex life and schedule is often life itself. I always hear patients say, "I would but I was tired." Exercise helps to remedy this in certain cases.

Journaling

Research has shown that journaling practices can ultimately result in a range of health benefits including a reduction of inflammation, the promotion of mental well-being, and even improved ventricular function. I often recommend journaling to my patients. It can be tricky in the context of pain, however. We don't want patients to put an ultra-focus on their symptoms or to perseverate about them, *but* it is also true that often in the process of treating pain we become so focused on the minutiae that we are unable to adequately see the strides we make. Journaling can help you keep a healthy perspective on things as you record the progress you make.

Journaling can be done in many ways, from a simple smiling face to sad face as you notice trends or patterns. Of course, you could actually jot down things you find helpful or frustrating in order to properly discuss and address those issues with your provider. Regardless, the benefits of journaling range from simply giving you a place to keep your thoughts organized to providing you with an outlet for reflection and self-expression. It's a practice I recommend and personally do myself!

Stress Management

This is a *big one!* Stress is everywhere, and it colors our lives in so many different ways.

Stress has a profoundly negative impact on the human microbiome, which has to do with the gut-brain axis. This concept is so important that it has been expanded to be called the microbiota-gut-brain axis. The communication is bidirectional—it is a gut-brain conversation. Stress also impacts our pelvic floors: When we are tense or stressed, our typical reaction is to "clench." And that clenching behavior undoubtedly occurs in our pelvic floors.

The result is that gut health, pelvic floor health, and brain health are linked. They are linked both in health and in dysfunction. The condition of your gut influences how you feel, how you present yourself, how motivated you are, and how your cognitive function operates. The condition of your brain also influences your microbial composition. If your brain gets involved in a stress response, it will pump out cortisol (one of the primary stress hormones) to help the body deal with danger. Because of the gastrointestinal link, it's a stress response you can actually feel—it's why you may feel "butterflies in your stomach" or a "nervous stomach" or experience stress-induced diarrhea. Because your pelvic floor is involved, you may even feel a burst of urinary symptoms like frequency, urgency, and even pain!

Believe it or not, this physiological mechanism can be seen in many neurological issues, including irritable bowel syndrome (often linked with anxiety and depression), pelvic floor dysfunction, interstitial cystitis, and inflammatory bowel disease. Our brains and bodies are built to communicate. Now let's hear them out!

Management of stress is not an easy thing. And navigating it is very individualized, as are the causes of stress. Often, just acknowledging the stress and admitting that it's playing a role in our lives is an important step for setting the stage for specific interventions.

Standing Desks

Sitting for long periods of time increases your risk of diabetes, heart disease, and early death. Whoa! It also affects your posture, shortens muscles, increases hypertonicity, and drastically affects the pelvic floor!

Standing desks are generally adjustable to your height, and believe it or not have been shown in recent studies to increase productivity. They are not suitable for everyone. For example, some doctors do not recommend standing desks for those who suffer from certain kinds of back pain or varicose veins. I often write prescriptions for standing desks for my patients who tend to sit for long periods of time. They have found using a standing desk helpful!

Vulvar Hygiene

Maintaining proper vulvar hygiene is important both for those who do and don't experience pain. The mainstream media tends to focus on skin care and frown line prevention, but why don't we give this same attention to pelvic and vaginal health? Let's start now.

Here are a few tips for maintaining vulvar hygiene:

- Avoid scented soaps, detergents, body washes, bath gels, and bubble baths.
- Wear nonconstricting cotton underwear during the day.
- Avoid pantyhose and tight pants.
- Use mild, hypoallergenic soap for bathing and only water for cleansing the vulva and vagina.
- Avoid douching, over-the-counter vaginal wipes, deodorants, and other commercial products.
- When necessary use unscented pads and tampons.
- Use a water-based, unscented, hypoallergenic lubricant for sex play.
- Avoid the use of fabric softener and dryer sheets on underwear.
- Apply ice or cold packs to the vulva for 10 to 15 minutes (up to six times per day) before and/or after sexual activity. To decrease deeper vaginal irritation, fill a glove with water and freeze it, then cut off only the finger portion and place it in the vagina. (It sounds crazy but it works.)
- Take warm baths twice a day with either Epsom salts or Aveeno oatmeal, which helps relieve irritation and itching.

Take-home point: There are many different lifestyle modifications that you can incorporate into your daily practices. Many of them can bring about drastic changes and improvements in our quality of life. It takes about 66 days to make something a habit, and habits affect your daily life. If you are experiencing pain, it is important to have the support of a physician who understands you and can help you navigate your symptoms, but it is also important for you to include habit-forming behaviors and rituals that support your efforts for wellness.

THE SCIENCE OF YOGA

Yoga is certainly in vogue in the United States. What's the science behind yoga, and how can yoga benefit patients with pelvic pain?

There are multiple physiologic benefits to yoga when practiced following the precautions listed later in this chapter. It:

- Calms and restores
- Decreases heart rate and respiratory rate
- Decreases blood pressure
- Decreases cortisol levels
- Increases blood flow to organs and intestines
- Decreases inflammatory markers
- Improves cell function
- Improves breath control
- Improves immune system function
- Reduces muscle tension

But one of the biggest benefits of practicing yoga, especially in regard to the pelvis, is that it lengthens and stretches muscles. This leads to reduced muscle tension and a reduction in chronic pain (including back and pelvic pain).

There are also many cognitive benefits to yoga; they include:

- Improves concentration
- Sharpens focus
- Increases mental clarity
- Increases ability to be present

This can and does translate to psychological (emotional and mental health) benefits:

- Reduces sleep disturbance
- Reduces anxiety and its negative effects
- Reduces depression
- Increases feelings of well-being
- Improves coping

The benefits of yoga on both the body and the mind have been well documented for thousands of years. More recent studies continue to support the idea that yoga, practiced correctly, can help to improve psychological well-being and to reduce pain symptoms. In a randomized study, 60 women with pelvic pain were divided into two groups: The first group received standard treatment with NSAIDs (nonsteroidal anti-inflammatory drugs) and the second group received yoga therapy in conjunction with standard treatment. After eight weeks of regular yoga practice (including asana, pranayama, and relaxation techniques), the second group saw a significant reduction in pain intensity and an improvement in physical, psychological, and social well-being.

As this study demonstrates, yoga can provide relief from chronic pelvic pain and thus contribute to a better overall quality of life. Additionally, yoga helps you connect with your physical body, which in turn can improve control over your pelvic floor and alleviate symptoms of pelvic floor dysfunction. Research shows that yoga may also reduce menstrual cramps and other pain symptoms associated with endometriosis.

Now let's get into some of the technical aspects of yoga that make it so therapeutic in so many ways.

Yoga and Breathing

Yoga has many health and wellness benefits. Individuals who suffer from pelvic pain can use yoga to help them decrease pain and to improve their quality of life. There are many different yoga methods and traditions, and most yoga practices include techniques for breathing, body positioning, and mindfulness to promote well-being. Technology allows individuals to use apps or websites to guide their yoga practice at home or at live instructed classes. This technology makes yoga widely accessible as a means of self-management of pelvic pain in conjunction with other treatments under the guidance of a health care provider.

Yoga commonly teaches deep breathing techniques, which are a helpful means to learn to relax and better coordinate the muscles of the pelvic floor. The ability to voluntarily relax your pelvic floor muscles helps you reduce pelvic pain by maintaining muscle mobility and proper circulation. The means by which breath work helps is both physiological and mechanical. When considering the role of breathing as it affects the pelvic floor, it is helpful to envision the trunk of the body as a house. In this paradigm, the respiratory diaphragm is the ceiling, the pelvic floor is the floor, and the abdominal and back muscles comprise the walls of the house. Thus, the pelvic floor muscles, diaphragm, and abdominal and spinal muscles must all work in symphony to stabilize the trunk, promote effective breathing, and maintain intra-abdominal pressure (IAP).

The diaphragm and pelvic floor work in a piston-like manner wherein as the diaphragm drops, drawing breath into the lungs during inhalation, the pelvic floor also drops. To expel air, it is vital that the diaphragm returns to its resting point and the pelvic floor lifts back up. This requires that the muscles maintaining the trunk are both strong and flexible. Thus, the abdominal and other core muscles are important in maintaining proper intra-abdominal pressure for breathing, posture, and bracing the spine during functional movements (as well as when you cough, sneeze, and have a bowel movement), and yoga can be a helpful practice in learning to better coordinate this symphony.

People who have had surgery, been pregnant, or have experienced chronic pelvic pain often exhibit shallow breathing. Restriction in one or more of these important muscles can cause a loss of coordination of the breathing muscles. This in turn can disrupt the piston-like mechanics of the diaphragm and pelvic floor, resulting in inefficient breathing and increased pressure on the pelvic floor.

Poses to Help Pelvic Pain

Yoga poses commonly used to assist those with pelvic pain include:

- Child's pose
- Happy baby
- Legs up the wall pose
- Garland pose (deep squat)

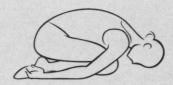

Child's pose

Precautions

As noted previously, some poses or types of yoga practice may not be suitable for you and, as with any new form of exercise, you should be sure to consult with your health care provider before starting yoga. For example, people who have excessive joint mobility, such as those with Ehlers-Danlos syndrome, should proceed with caution when beginning a yoga program. Yoga poses often involve placing the body into a stretch, and some poses are held for more than a minute. Placing excessive stretch on the joints, tendons, and ligaments in people with hypermobile joints and soft tissue can in some cases cause more harm than good. The same goes for those with back pain, hip or shoulder issues, and pregnant women, among others who should consult with their health care provider before starting a yoga program.

Be sure to find a yoga instructor who has education and knowledge of your condition. For example, a sign of a good instructor in an in-person class is one who circulates around the room to ensure that participants are demonstrating correct alignment and safe postures, versus one who remains at the front of the class the entire time.

Some yoga poses place the body in extreme end-of-range positions, and when not performed properly, aggravation or even injury to a joint can result.

Some examples of these extreme poses include:

- Pigeon pose
- Wheel
- Headstand
- Shoulder stand
- Hero pose
- Forward bend (can be harmful if knees are locked)

It is advised that a skilled instructor be present when attempting any of these poses.

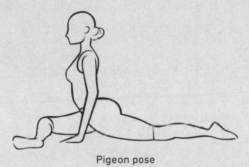

Pigeon pose

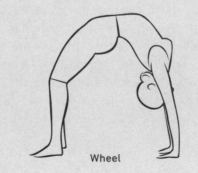

Wheel

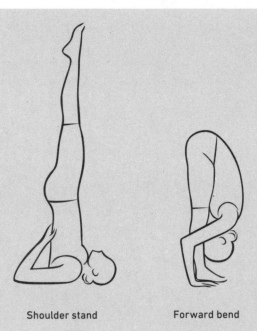

Shoulder stand   Forward bend

Be Gracious with Yourself

A quiet, meditative yoga practice can work wonders for some people and can invoke anxiety for others. It is important to recognize that some people will benefit more from other forms of exercise if they are not yet ready for the pensive and quiet nature of yoga. The beauty of yoga is that there are many different types of yoga practices, and it can be fun to try new forms to see which suits your body and personality best. Ultimately, some people will benefit more from a breathing exercise practice while walking in a beautiful area, while swimming, or performing other forms of body movement. Give yourself grace if you are struggling with a yoga practice and invite yourself to try other things—you never know what you might find that truly allows you to relax and become mindful!

Case Study: Josh

JOSH was suffering from weakening erections. At the age of 32, it was something he couldn't wrap his head around. He worried it would happen every time he was put in a position to perform. To compound that fear, more recently he noticed he was developing pain at the tip of the penis after erections. In addition, Josh was experiencing other pain, especially in his coccyx and pelvic region. He worked as a computer programmer, meaning he sat for long hours at a time coding.

Before he came to me, he had seen a urologist who prescribed Cialis, which he thought was giving him relief from the pain at the tip of his penis, but he realized after months that not much had changed. Josh was a huge CrossFitter in his time off, but he had to take a break from this because after his workouts his pain would increase. His anxiety starting catapulting him through the roof. He was unable to go out with his friends. He was scared to engage in sexual activity. And now the one activity that gave him stress relief was increasing his pain. He was distraught when he got to my office.

"Dr. Bahlani . . . I've been on rounds of antibiotics. I've changed my daily lifestyle. I've stopped exercising. Nothing has been working! The only thing that helps me is if I have a small glass of vodka at night. What is wrong with me?"

We sat down and discussed goals. They were simple. Josh wanted his life back. His exam revealed a heightened sphincter tone with an immense amount of hypertonicity and pain surrounding the prostate. Josh had undiagnosed category IIIB CP/CPPS (chronic prostatitis/chronic pelvic pain). As I do with many of my patients, we started with intense pelvic floor physical therapy and local muscle relaxants.

In six weeks, Josh was sitting through work without pain. He had also gotten a standing desk, which helped. He had much less pain after ejaculations and noticed better quality erections. He was happy. But he wasn't out of the woods yet. He wanted to try coming off his muscle relaxant suppository. He wanted to restart CrossFit. He wanted to be able to carve out less time for physical therapy. We decided to move forward with a pudendal nerve block to bathe the nerve with anti-inflammatory and anesthetics and Botox to the levator ani complex surrounding the prostate.

Within four weeks of the procedure, Josh was back to his CrossFit workouts, was tapering off his medication, and was going to physical therapy only once every two weeks. He was having "a lot of sex" that was pain-free and pleasurable, and he finally felt like he understood his issues enough to prevent their recurrence.

And while I don't see Josh anymore, I recently received photos of his engagement and he couldn't be happier. This is what it is all about!

13

ALTERNATIVE TREATMENTS

A s with the other possible treatments that your health care provider may recommend, please be sure to follow any specific guidance they may have given you about the alternative treatments I'll discuss here.

ACUPUNCTURE

Acupuncture techniques date back almost 3,000 years. During this time, it has not only survived but also grown in popularity, which is a testament to its value. Acupuncture uses specialized needles to stimulate specific points along important channels within our bodies. Approximately 400 acupuncture points, or acupoints, are located along various channels (also known as meridians). Acupuncture comes to us through traditional Chinese medicine (TCM), which is one of the most ancient branches of medicine in the world. TCM comprises many forms of treatment, including acupuncture, cupping, herbal medicine, massage, exercise, and diet therapy. TCM is based on the belief that the body's vital energy (qi) circulates through the meridians, which create a network of pathways connected to our organs and their functions.

I'm a huge fan of acupuncture, as it embodies the concept of ancient healing medicine as a combination of both science and art, which has taken millennia to develop. It differs markedly from modern allopathic medicine; in acupuncture, the treatment for the particular presenting complaint, for example pelvic pain, may have variations due to the emotional, physical, and other pathology present in the patient. In other words, no two individuals who present with similar complaints are necessarily given the same acupuncture treatment. It is this unique individuality of treatment that has made acupuncture a powerful technique in the hands of experienced practitioners of the art. It is also this unique individuality that makes acupuncture extremely difficult to study, as it often lacks reproducibility.

Acupuncture has been applied to a number of acute and chronic medical conditions, such as pain, male and female sexual dysfunction, pregnancy, related physiologic changes, cardiovascular disorders, asthma, sports-related injuries, and cancer treatment–related side effects. Acupuncture has also gained significant support for its role in pain management, including in the field of chronic pelvic pain.

The mechanism by which acupuncture affects pain is not accurately understood yet. Traditionally, the thought was that qi, the energy of life, was manipulated by activating various acupoints along the meridians. Acupuncture, therefore, is used to help restore the flow of qi through the meridians.

When applied to neuromuscular issues related to pelvic pain, the practice of needling these tightened areas or trigger points can be helpful for the release and resolution of symptoms. Acupuncture has also been thought to be helpful in decreasing inflammation, again another important aspect in the treatment of pelvic pain syndromes.

Many people turn to acupuncture for their pelvic health issues. Although many of us allopathic physicians argue that needling itself has helpful healing properties, especially when done in conjunction with medications like nerve blocks or Botox, one cannot argue with the fact that dry needling in the form of acupuncture has been used for centuries.

Will Acupuncture Help My Pelvic Pain?

This is a question I get asked relatively frequently. The short answer is yes; there are studies that have looked at acupuncture in relation to pelvic pain. And guess what? It has been shown to be helpful.

Often, you may see that traditional therapies (by that I mean oral medications or certain types of injections or compounded medications) have become the gold standard when treating pelvic pain. That happened for a reason: In most cases, traditional therapies have been proven to provide effective relief from pain symptoms. However, no two cases of pelvic pain are alike. While one person may respond well to traditional therapies, another will struggle to find relief, even after trying every known trick in the book. This is when it may be time to turn to alternative therapies for pelvic pain.

Why? Because staying on the cutting edge of current health trends is what pushes the field forward. I want the best for my patients, and I believe it's my duty to offer the very best pain management techniques.

Sometimes this means stepping away from the traditional route and considering alternative treatment options, such as acupuncture, cannabidiol (CBD) products, yoga, or various types of cognitive or behavioral therapy. These therapies are believed to provide relief from pelvic pain. That said, when dealing with alternative therapies, it's a constant challenge to know for sure whether they're safe and effective or not, but the medical community has done the research and is there to help you make the best decisions for your health.

In a treatment such as acupuncture, the needles are inserted into specific acupressure points to stimulate certain organs and release qi. There is no scientific proof for TCM concepts, such as qi and acupuncture points. However, current research shows that acupuncture may provide some relief from chronic pain. The research has been so strong, in fact, that the National Institutes of Health (NIH) has said that acupuncture appears to be a viable treatment option for those with chronic pain conditions. Other studies have noted that acupuncture can be effective in treating pelvic pain when used in conjunction with traditional methods.

What Other Conditions Can Be Treated Using Acupuncture?

For women, data shows that acupuncture can improve fertility. Studies have shown that acupuncture increases the effectiveness of fertility treatments and medications by naturally raising the hormone levels that travel to the ovaries. This is of particular importance for people with polycystic ovarian syndrome (PCOS). Acupuncture has also been shown to balance hormones and therefore to regulate ovulation, which may increase the chances of successful pregnancy by 33 percent.

For men, acupuncture may provide relief from prostatitis. Several small studies suggest that acupuncture can have a positive impact on prostatitis pain. In the studies, men who received acupuncture treatments saw a significant reduction in symptoms compared to men who received a placebo or no acupuncture.

In essence, the mechanism by which acupuncture is thought to be helpful is uncertain and varies from source to source. However, it should be noted that acupuncture has been studied in many different conditions and subjectively the data appears to show benefits.

How Does One Choose a Good Acupuncturist?

Get referrals. The popularity of acupuncture has grown tremendously over the past few years. Chances are, you can find someone in your social circle who has tried it. Seeking out recommendations, especially from someone who has seen an acupuncturist for reasons similar to your own, can help you understand the procedure and narrow down the practitioner's clinical strength and niche. This in turn can accelerate progress and symptom relief.

Expertise. In acupuncture, as with allopathic medicine, treating some conditions requires more experience and training than others. Pain, fertility, cancer, and dermatological conditions can be particularly complicated issues to treat with acupuncture and are often best handled by specialists with a particular niche or expertise. There are numerous ways an acupuncturist might amass this type of experience, including certification courses, extra training via apprenticeships or fellowships, or simply a high patient load in that area due to their clinical interest. One way or another, finding a specialist makes a big difference.

Facilities matter. From what I've seen with my patients' experiences, the best results occur in an environment that breeds relaxation and stress relief. Acupuncture offices vary widely. Some are small and quaint. Others are clinical and perhaps very "medical or sterile." Some are grandiose and spa-like. Ask yourself what environment you feel most comfortable in. If there are no photos on the websites or literature you consult, consider dropping by the facility to see if it's a good fit!

Personal preference. Finding a good acupuncturist is like finding a good partner. I mean that. It's important to create a healing relationship that fits with the values and ideals you feel are important. It's important that the relationship be therapeutic, much like a collaborative partnership. This is the key that often sets apart those who find acupuncture helpful versus those who don't find it to be much help.

WANDS AND DILATORS

Pelvic health tools such as dilators and pelvic wands can help empower people to manage their pelvic pain. These tools may be used as a component of a home self-care program in tandem with formalized pelvic physical therapy, and in some cases they may be used independently, always following the advice of your health care professional. Both tools help empower people to treat their pelvic pain and to help them reach their goal of performing various life tasks again.

How to Treat Deep Pelvic Floor Pain Using the Pelvic Wand

As previously mentioned, conditions of chronic pelvic pain are often caused by overactivity or tightness in the pelvic floor muscles. As many as one in seven people suffer from chronic pelvic pain, and they often spend years trying to receive a proper explanation and diagnosis for their pain. The pelvic floor muscles can become tight or restricted for various reasons. In some instances, the restriction in the pelvic floor muscles is caused by poor posture, a fall, injury, surgery, or emotional trauma resulting in clenching of the muscles. Stress can cause people to clench the pelvic floor in a reflexive guarding manner, leading to tender points in the pelvic floor muscles. Trigger points, which are also known as tender points, are characterized by the presence of taut bands or "knots" in the muscle, as well as the generation of a referral pattern of pain. Trigger points are areas of tenderness occurring in the muscles, muscle-tendon junctions, bursa, or fat pads. They are commonly present in chronic pelvic pain conditions that include vaginismus, vestibulodynia, vulvodynia, coccygeus, proctalgia fugax, and endometriosis. Trigger points may also occur after childbirth and following pelvic surgery, such as a hysterectomy.

The good news is that it is possible to release the pelvic floor muscles by performing gentle stretches, learning to relax the muscles on command, and using a pelvic wand.

Common symptoms of pelvic pain due to trigger points or tender points include:

- Aching sensation from deep inside the pelvis
- Burning sensations around the bladder or while urinating (without a bacterial infection)
- Sexual pain with no known cause
- Inability to tolerate vaginal penetration for sex, medical exams, or tampon use
- Pain in the tailbone (coccyx)
- Chronic constipation with an unknown cause
- Pain in the groin
- Abdomen pain

Retraining the pelvic floor muscles to relax takes time. Many people who endure chronic pelvic pain had experienced abuse, rape, surgery, radiation, or a traumatic event that preceded their pelvic pain. For this reason, counseling may be beneficial while working on training the body. Anxiety, stress, pain, as well as the fear of pain often reinforce the symptoms of chronic pelvic pain. The process of healing involves learning to sense when the muscles are about to spasm and then training the brain to relax them prior to when the contractions start.

Treatment of Deep Pelvic Floor Muscle Tension

A pelvic wand can allow you to release painful trigger points in the pelvic floor. The unique ergonomic design of a pelvic wand allows you to reach the hard-to-reach muscles of the pelvic floor for relief. To decrease pelvic pain caused by trigger points, the keys to success, based on the experiences of my patients, are the consistent use of the pelvic wand and the practice of pelvic floor muscle relaxation prior to or after wand use. Trigger point release, coupled with relaxation techniques and focused attention on training the muscles, are both components of reducing deep pelvic floor muscle tension.

As with any new health care practice, you should consult with a health care provider before using the pelvic wand. Your health care provider may have a unique training plan for you outside of the recommendations made here.

How to Use the Pelvic Wand

General use of the wand includes sessions that consist of a 15- to 30-minute breathing exercise and wand use at least three times per week for as long as needed to relieve ongoing pain. A pelvic wand can be used daily as needed.

1. Wash the wand with warm water and soap.
2. Designate a place in your home that is safe, quiet, and comfortable, such as your bed.
3. Decide which end of the wand to use. The long, thin end is beneficial for the deeper pelvic floor muscles, whereas the shorter rounded end is for the muscles near the entrance of the vagina or to address tender points in the rectum.
4. Use a generous amount of water-based lubricant on the first 1 to 2 inches of the desired treatment end of the wand, as well as on the opening of the vagina. The use of a water-based lubricant is important to preserve the medical-grade silicone of the wand.

5. Start by lying on your back with knees bent and resting on pillows for support. Some people may prefer to lie on their side instead. If that's the case, be sure to bend your knees and to support your top leg with a folded pillow between your knees.

6. Begin your session by breathing in and allowing your belly to expand, followed by exhaling, allowing your belly to slowly fall. The act of slowly exhaling helps to naturally relax the pelvic floor muscles. Repeat the deep-breathing pattern and continue to do so steadily and deliberately. Gently bring the wand to the opening of the vagina and carefully insert it at approximately ½ to 1 inch (if this is your first time). Continue breathing and insert to greater depths as you feel comfortable—for most people the superficial muscles are at a depth of approximately 1 inch, while the deeper muscles are at a depth of 4 to 6 inches.

7. Gently sweep the end of the wand until you encounter a tender point. When you find a tender point, gently compress the end of the wand into the tender point with the same firmness you would use to check a tomato for ripeness. Do not press so hard you squish the tomato.

8. Maintain gentle pressure on the tender point and slowly move your bent knee left and right until you find a position that stops the pain in the pelvic floor muscle. When you find this position, remain there for one to two minutes to allow the tender point to fully release. Continue to breathe deeply.

9. Repeat this process one or two times per day or as needed.

Vaginal Dilators (Trainers) as a Tool for Overcoming Painful Penetration

Vaginal dilators, also referred to as vaginal trainers, are used to restore vaginal width, depth, and elasticity to allow for sexual activity, tampon use, or medical exams. They commonly are sold in sets or individually and are made of plastic or silicone. They are usually cylinder shaped with a tapered end, and gradually get longer and wider in size. They are commonly recommended for people with conditions including vaginismus, muscle spasms around the opening of the vagina, menopause-related vaginal atrophy, postpartum scar tissue pain, and gender affirming procedures. Additionally, they are commonly prescribed after certain types of cancer treatments such as radiation, chemotherapy, and surgery. They are also indicated for use for those with genetic conditions of vaginal agenesis such as Mayer-Rokitansky-Küster-Hauser (MRKH) syndrome and androgen insensitivity syndrome (AIS). Furthermore, they are indicated for use by people with vestibulodynia and vulvodynia for desensitization therapy.

Keys to Successful Vaginal Training for Vaginismus and Vaginal Pain

Vaginismus treatment can include the use of vaginal dilators while learning to relax the pelvic floor muscles. Based on the experiences of my patients, to decrease pain with vaginal penetration, the keys to success are consistency and routine practice. Daily use of dilators for 10 to 30 minutes per session, coupled with relaxation techniques and focused attention on training the muscles to relax, should result in reducing vaginal pain with vaginal penetration.

Always consult with a health care provider before starting a new training plan, and using a vaginal dilator is no different. Your health care provider may have a unique training plan for you that is different from the recommendations made here, and you should follow that tailored plan.

How to Start Using Vaginal Dilators

Choosing a dilator set can be intimidating. There is a misconception that dilators "stretch" the vagina. The vaginal canal naturally stretches as exemplified by its ability to accommodate a penis or a baby's head. The purpose of dilators is to desensitize the vaginal muscles and nervous system to the sensation of penetration. Working with dilators will train the pelvic floor and nervous system to feel safe and comfortable with penetration—quieting the limbic systemic response, resulting in involuntary pelvic muscle spasms.

1. Select a vaginal trainer recommended by your health care provider.
2. Wash the dilator with warm water and soap.
3. Designate a place in your home that is safe and comfortable for your vaginal trainer practice. Choose a place that is quiet and calming.
4. Use a generous amount of water-based lubricant on the vaginal trainer and the opening of the vagina. The use of a water-based lubricant is important to preserve the medical-grade silicone of the vaginal trainer.
5. Start by lying on your back with your knees bent and feet planted. Some people may prefer to lie on their side instead; if

that's the case, be sure to have your knees bent and the top leg supported by a folded pillow between your knees.

6. Begin your training by breathing in and allowing your belly to expand, followed by exhaling and allowing your belly to slowly fall. The act of slowly exhaling can naturally open the vagina. Repeat the deep-breathing pattern and continue to do so steadily and deliberately. Gently bring the vaginal trainer to the opening of the vagina and carefully insert it.

7. Keep the vaginal trainer inserted in the vagina and repeat the slow, deep breathing cycle for 10 to 30 minutes (or the length of time recommended by your health care provider, if different). Some people benefit from practicing for 10 minutes three times daily.

8. If you experience discomfort, visual imagery is helpful for relaxing the pelvic floor muscles around the opening of the vagina. There are several images that can work. Pick the one that is best for you: "Imagine that the vagina is like a rose, blooming outward and opening"; "Imagine that the vagina is like an umbrella, opening and expanding"; or "Imagine that the vagina is like an elastic band, flexible and mobile."

9. Repeat this process daily and progress to larger trainers as you are able and according to your goals.

DEEP BREATHING FOR PELVIC PAIN

Learning to breathe properly is an important part of healing pelvic and vaginal pain. Many people with pelvic pain have limited breathing. Learning to breathe and expand the rib cage and abdomen helps to improve overall circulation, reduce strain on the pelvic floor muscles, and reduce tension in the neck, head, and shoulders.

Breath practice can include the following daily basic exercise. Follow these simple steps to begin:

- Find a comfortable position lying down. Often, it is helpful to put pillows or a bolster under the knees to reduce tension in the lower back.
- Place one hand on the breastbone and the other on the stomach. The goal during this breathing exercise is to keep the chest still but allow the stomach to rise and fall with the breath.
- Breathe in slowly and deeply through the nose, allowing your stomach to gently rise, keeping the chest still.
- Exhale gently through the mouth, allowing the stomach to gently fall. Pay close attention to your stomach rising and falling as you breathe in through the nose and out through the mouth.
- Continue to take nice, slow breaths as you allow all thoughts and disruptions to fade away. Visualize the tension in your body being released as your body relaxes.

Breathing with a Body Scan or Reduced Tension

Learning to detect when you are clenching your muscles takes practice initially, because often the brain is occupied with the stressor or task at hand and is not privy to the fact that the muscles are overactive.

Body scanning is an exercise to better detect the sensation of clenched muscles, thus training the brain to coordinate and release them.

To start, find a comfortable position lying down. Often it is helpful to put pillows or a bolster under the knees to reduce tension in the low back. Place one hand on the breastbone, and the other on the stomach. The goal during this breathing exercise is to keep the chest still, and to allow the stomach to expand and fall with the breath.

Breathe in slowly and deeply through the nose and imagine that the rib cage is an umbrella, expanding in all directions outward as you inhale. Then exhale gently through the mouth as the rib cage and stomach gently returns down. Continue to take easy breaths as you allow all thoughts and disruptions to fade away. Visualize the tension in your body being released as your body relaxes.

Practice releasing tension in the body and specifically in the pelvic floor muscles and the muscles around the vagina. To do this, begin by focusing attention on the feet. The feet share common nerves with the pelvic floor, so it is helpful to practice noticing the muscles in the feet clenching and unclenching. Take note of any tension in the feet and allow them to unclench and relax.

Next, do the same with your gluteal muscles. Maintain your breathing, do not hold your breath, and unclench the gluteal muscles if they are tense.

Now, bring your attention to your abdominal muscles. Keep breathing and release tension in the abdomen as you inhale and allow the rib cage to expand like an umbrella.

Finally, notice the tension around the shoulders, neck, and jaw. Maintain your breathing and release the shoulders from your ears if they are elevated, unclench your jaw, and allow your tongue to rest.

This method of body scanning is helpful in learning to sense when the muscles are involuntarily active. Over time this notic-ing will result in less overall load on the muscles, which is helpful in returning them to a healthier and better coordinated state for improved functioning.

HOW TO UTILIZE BREATH WORK

Can your breathing patterns be affecting your pelvic pain?

This is probably a question most of you never even thought to ask. The answer, however, may surprise you: yes. Don't forget, treat-ing pelvic pain involves a multifactorial approach. There are a great deal of basic lifestyle modifications that can have tremendous down-stream effects on pelvic pain. Two different studies demonstrated that patients suffering from pelvic pain often practice faulty breathing pat-terns. This means that correcting faulty breathing patterns may really benefit you.

If you breathe mostly in your upper chest, it can lead to decreased lower lateral rib excursion, which in turn causes increased muscle tone in your abdominals. This increased intra-abdominal pressure can cause increased stress on the pelvic floor.

Paradoxical relaxation therapy, a daily practice that seeks to culti-vate effortlessness in the presence of pain and tension, can help to relax the shortened muscles in the pelvic floor. Also known as the Wise-Anderson Protocol or Standford pelvic pain protocol, this therapy is very accessible in the book *Paradoxical Relaxation: Dissolving Anxi-ety by Accepting It*, by David Wise, and often implemented in specific pelvic floor physical therapy programs.

In addition, most of us hold our breath often or breathe shallowly, taking anxious, short breaths. Deep, slow, full breaths have a profound effect on resetting the stress response because of activation of the vagus nerve, which promotes relaxation. The vagus nerve goes through your diaphragm and is activated with every deep breath.

Pro-tip: Make your exhales longer than your inhales. Inhale for four counts then increase the exhale for five or six counts. This will help activate your vagus nerve and slow down your heart rate.

Understanding this relationship and incorporating seemingly simple lifestyle modifications can bring life-altering changes. Take a moment today to notice your own breathing patterns. It starts with the basics!

Other ways in which breathing can affect your pain? Let's discuss it further.

The Vagus Nerve (no reference to Las Vegas)

The vagus nerve is the longest of the cranial nerves. It has more than 100,000 fibers and communicates bidirectionally between the brain and parts of our bodies. Many refer to the vagus nerve as the information superhighway, with 80 percent of the fibers communicating from the body to the brain and the other 20 percent communicating from the brain to the body.

The vagus nerve activates the parasympathetic nervous system, which is also called the rest and digest system. A big part of the vagus nerve's job is to tell the brain what is happening in your organs. The vagus nerve is also vital for calming the body after a stressful moment, as it works to help bring your body out of "fight or flight" mode. If you have poor vagal tone, it can stop your body from going into the "rest and digest" mode.

Symptoms of poor vagal tone include:

- Digestive issues, including symptoms of IBS or SIBO
- Pelvic floor or pelvic pain issues (including urinary changes and bowel pattern changes)
- Anxiety or depression
- Upper chest breathing (short, quick breaths)
- High blood pressure
- Changes in heart rate (racing or decreased)
- Insomnia
- Feelings of inability to rest
- Chronic muscle tension

Vagus nerve impairment is related to both pelvic pain and jaw pain, believe it or not! Here's an example: When the jaw isn't aligned, say through a condition such as TMJ, the trigeminal nerve is aggravated. The fibers of the trigeminal nerve connect with the fibers of the vagus nerve inside the brain, meaning when the trigeminal nerve is overstimulated the vagus nerve is impacted.

They work kind of like a seesaw action—the trigeminal nerve is associated with the sympathetic nervous system and the vagus nerve is associated with the parasympathetic nervous system.

This is the exact mechanism thought to be involved in many pelvic pain disorders involving the pudendal nerve. The pudendal nerve has both motor and sensory functions. Many causes of pelvic pain disorders can anatomically and mechanically disrupt or irritate the pudendal nerve, which thereby again can affect the vagus nerve.

Having the ability to activate the vagus nerve and to increase vagal tone can be central to keeping the pelvic floor and TMJ (they are related) at bay!

> SIDE NOTE: How are TMJ and pelvic floor dysfunction related? Think about it this way: When you are stressed or tense, do you ever notice yourself clenching your jaw? Many people, in fact, clench their pelvic floors, as well. Studies show that many people who suffer from pelvic pain disorders also suffer from TMJ! The more you know, right?!

How to Activate the Vagus Nerve

3D diaphragmatic breathing: By slowing down and focusing on your breath (long, deep excursions of the diaphragm), you alter the way your brain stem signals the diaphragm to contract.

Movement: By moving your body, you help decrease compression and irritation of the nerves (both trigeminal and pudendal), and this increases vagal tone.

Sing and laugh: Believe it or not, singing and laughing increases beta-endorphins, nitric oxide, and capillary blood flow. The combined effect benefits the entire vascular system while boosting vagal tone.

Hot-cold plunges: Submersions into hot then cold water help stimulate the vagus nerve, thereby decreasing sympathetic activation and increasing vagal tone.

Breath Work for Life

The truth is that breathing is extremely important to how our bodies function overall. If our breathing patterns are faulty and nonfunctional, then all our movements will follow in tow. There are many reasons for this, but specifically, different phases of inhalation and exhalation are intrinsically coupled with certain muscular and joint movements. For instance, when we "breathe in" the spine extends, the pelvis tilts forward, and the arms and shoulders externally rotate. Conversely, when we "breathe out" the spine flexes, the pelvis tilts underneath, and the arms and shoulders internally rotate. For some (I actually would argue that for many), this biomechanical interplay is not actually functioning correctly. The downstream effects of this malfunctioning include compensatory behaviors that increase chronic muscle tension and neuropathic upregulation that's often related to chronic pain.

In this sense, the restoration of proper breathing mechanics can be life altering in a sense.

CANNABIDIOL (CBD)

As you can probably see by now, treating pain is . . . complex. Unfortunately, traditional medicine can often leave those suffering with a great deal of unmet needs and unanswered questions. This requires us, as clinicians, to understand the role of nonconventional methods in patient care, CBD being one product that has quickly gained popularity among many health care professionals in our patients' treatment plans. You should speak with your health care provider before using CBD for treatment of your pelvic pain.

CBD for medical use has been getting a whole lot of media buzz in recent years. New CBD manufacturers are appearing all the time, and cannabis stores are seemingly cropping up on every corner. It's easy to get caught up in the hype and believe that CBD is the magical cure-all we've all been waiting for. But how much of the hype is actually true?

Research is still in its infancy, and there's a lot we still don't know about CBD, particularly as it relates to treating pelvic pain. To break down the myth about CBD and its mystical healing properties, let's start with what we know for sure about this elusive compound:

- CBD is a nonpsychoactive compound found in marijuana and hemp. In other words, it's the part of marijuana that doesn't get you high but is believed to provide a host of health-promoting benefits.
- CBD has been shown to effectively treat some types of epilepsy. For example, recent studies have shown that CBD can be used in the treatment of severe childhood epilepsy syndromes that typically don't respond to anti-seizure medications, reducing, or even eliminating, seizures in some patients with these conditions. In fact, CBD has been shown to be so effective against severe forms of epilepsy that the FDA recently approved the first cannabis-derived epilepsy medication.
- CBD can prevent insomnia. Believe it or not, the connection between CBD and sleep dates back to around 1200 A.D., when it was mentioned in an ancient Chinese medical text.

Modern studies also show that CBD may help you fall asleep and stay asleep.

- CBD may help alleviate anxiety. A number of studies have shown that there is a link between CBD and anxiety, but many researchers attribute this to the placebo effect. Basically, these studies show that if you believe CBD will reduce anxiety, it will, regardless of any real scientific effect.
- CBD may help treat chronic pain. Various studies have explored the relationship between CBD and chronic pain conditions, including arthritis and inflammatory and neuropathic pain. These studies suggest that CBD may help lower or inhibit pain and inflammation, but further research is needed before we can fully understand the connection and the side effects and potential risks.

CBD for medical use is currently unregulated, and critics of CBD warn about its safety. Because CBD is considered a supplement and not a drug, it isn't subject to the same federal regulations as traditional medications. Doses vary from product to product, and the most effective therapeutic dose of CBD is unknown, which can make it confusing (and potentially harmful) for people to use it as part of their treatment plan. As noted, it's important to speak with a medical professional before you start to use a CBD product to treat pelvic pain (or any health condition).

Will CBD Help My Bladder?

It is truly a question I get on a daily basis. The truth is, the jury is still out. And right now there's not yet enough data for me to unwaveringly say, yes!

However, I think it's important to note that to date, multiple studies (one of which was a randomized controlled multicenter clinical trial) have been conducted suggesting that there are cannabinoid receptors in the bladder. This begs for further exploration of the analgesic and antispasmodic properties of phytocannabinoids in patients with voiding dysfunction and bladder pain. It's a topic I find super interesting, and I believe it deserves a great deal of further investigation.

We can extrapolate this concept a bit further to investigate whether CBD can be helpful in other pelvic pain syndromes, including pelvic floor dysfunction, vulvodynia or vestibulodynia, interstitial cystitis, and endometriosis.

But we won't get ahead of ourselves. There's a lot we still don't know about these nontraditional methods, even if there is increasing evidence that they could be an effective complement to a holistic pain treatment plan.

Frequent Questions and Answers Regarding CBD and Pain

Even though the research is still in early stages, why do you believe in CBD's potential to be prescribed for pain in the future?
I love this question: It implies the understanding that everything in medicine is essentially a ratio of risk versus benefit. One aspect of our

jobs as physicians is to weigh these risks and benefits (especially in the setting of alternative therapies with premature evidence) on a case-by-case basis to see what works best for each individual.

That having been said, studies suggest that CBD for medical use (in its various forms) generally has a low side-effect profile (that is, CBD alone is not considered to be psychoactive) and may be a relatively low-risk adjunctive treatment option with the potential to be used in a wide variety of treatment applications. Patients suffering from pain can often feel frustrated with treatment options, with neuro-modulating medications and opioids coming with their own significant risk-benefit ratio. If formulations of CBD could help wean people off other medications or even act as a first-line treatment option prior to more addictive alternatives, I think there is good reason to further explore CBD as an effective strategy.

There are so many different types of CBD (tinctures, topical balms, gel caps); how do I know which is the best for me?
This is a tough one because there is such little data on absorption and effectivity rates of CBD, which in turn vary depending on dose and preparation. In addition, variables like where the CBD was grown and the type of CBD itself can have an effect on its medicinal qualities. For example, a tincture of CBD drops may be different and variable depending on each product and company. A dose can range anywhere from 3 mg to 50 mg. This also holds true for CBD balms. Remember, while there are cannabinoid receptors in many areas of our bodies, absorption and effectivity rates vary depending on dose and preparation. It is imperative that you discuss different products and methods of administration/absorption with your physician to help figure out which type would be the best for you.

———

Is there a possibility that CBD can have an intoxicating or mental-status altering effect?

CBD alone is thought to contain at maximum 0.3% THC. THC is believed to have psychoactive properties while CBD alone is not thought to harbor enough to cause psychoactive changes. The issue that arises is related to the fact that CBD supplements are not well regulated. One way to combat this is to ask the seller for a Certificate of Analysis (COA). Many people are unaware of the importance of asking for this. A COA provides the buyer with a breakdown of what is in the product and more specifically if it contains any sort of heavy metals, pesticides, or harmful contaminants. If a CBD product you're considering doesn't have a COA, it may be best to choose another product.

CBD and Sex: What's Up with CBD Lubricants?

Let's get right down to business: CBD can be used to improve your sex life. Yes, you read that right. Cannabis-based products, such as CBD lubricants, can have positive effects far beyond getting high. We've all heard that CBD can help with stress, insomnia, or pain—but recent studies show that CBD can also be used to spice things up between the sheets.

The Link between CBD and Sex

Before using any CBD product, during sex or otherwise, you should consult with your health care professional and follow their advice. If CBD is part of your treatment plan, it's important to understand that CBD is not regulated by the FDA. It is treated as a dietary supplement, not a medication, so doses vary greatly from product to product. It's always best to err on the side of caution and to start small to get an idea of how your body tolerates CBD. Once you have a better idea of how CBD affects you (and your sex life), you can work your way up from there if desired (following your health care provider's tailored guidance, of course).

As for how CBD affects your sex life, a recent survey showed that 68 percent of people who used a CBD product during sex found that it improved their sex life. The study also showed that, unfortunately, a whopping 96 percent of people have no idea that CBD can have benefits during sex and more than half don't know that CBD can be used for sex at all.

But the research shows that there are actually many benefits of using CBD during sex. Here's how:

- CBD can reduce anxiety. It's long been believed that CBD can curb stress and anxiety, so it stands to reason, and confirmed by research, that it can also help with performance anxiety.
- CBD can help to decrease inflammation and potentially alleviate pelvic pain. CBD also helps to relax your muscles, which can be especially helpful for those suffering from certain pelvic pain disorders.
- Personal CBD lubricants may enhance sexual desire and pleasure by increasing blood flow to your genitals. This can increase stimulation, sensation, and arousal.

Sounds pretty good, right? Keep reading to find out how to use CBD during sex, if it's part of your treatment plan.

How to Use CBD in the Bedroom

So how does CBD come into play during sex? You can introduce CBD into your sex life in so many ways! Lubricants, tinctures, oral gels, sprays . . . there are many different types of CBD-based sex products you can try to see which works for you. CBD lubricants can be especially powerful during sex, particularly for those looking to increase sensation or to reduce pelvic pain. Here are some tips for choosing a safe, effective CBD lube:

- Check the ingredient list. All CBD lubricants are not created equally. Some contain harmful or irritating products, such as sugars or alcohols, that may lead to infection. Always read the ingredient list before buying or using any CBD lube to make sure you're putting only safe products on your most sensitive areas! I would recommend staying away from products that contain things like parabens, sulfates, and propylene glycol.
- Choose water-based CBD lube and avoid oil-based products. Oil-based CBD lubes can break down the latex in condoms, which is problematic for obvious reasons. CBD oil itself can cause the same issue, so it's important to pick a water-based CBD lube that's specifically made for sex.
- Buy CBD lube from a reputable company. Just like you should use only the best quality skin care products or eat the highest quality food, you should use only CBD products that come from reputable sources. Do your research to find the best CBD lubricant you can. You may need to try a few before you find the right one for you.

While there are no guaranteed benefits of CBD for sex, there's strong evidence that CBD can be a positive addition to your sex life by easing anxiety and improving sexual function. At the very least, it's always fun to try something new in the bedroom. And if you get a little extra pleasure out of it, then that's a bonus!

———————

When it comes to CBD and pelvic pain, there are a lot of unknowns. At the end of the day, only time and continued research will tell if CBD can help with pain treatment. But even though the research isn't definitive, there's also increasing evidence that CBD can treat conditions of many kinds, including chronic pain and inflammation.

For now, we know that an estimated 50 million Americans suffer from chronic pain, and approximately 15 percent of women (and 3 to 6 percent of men) will experience chronic pelvic pain at some point in their lives. It's clear that pain has become an epidemic and traditional medicine isn't giving people the relief they deserve, leaving many with unmet needs, unanswered questions, and avenues of exploration for alternative remedies—such as CBD.

PROBIOTICS, PREBIOTICS, AND THE MICROBIOME

Probiotics are live microorganisms that confer health benefits. And there certainly is a large market for probiotics for genitourinary health. Do these particular probiotics work? Unfortunately, the data isn't clear-cut. Studies that look at probiotic use for bacterial vaginosis and vulvovaginal candidiasis (yeast infection) have been mixed, meaning some experience benefits while others don't appear to benefit much.

———————

Studies that combine and analyze the data of multiple studies (meta-analyses) have also been mixed, some showing benefits and others not. One meta-analysis study in 2020 showed that probiotics used as a supplement to conventional anti-yeast or antibiotic treatment for bacterial vaginosis (BV) and yeast infections are effective in the short term (less than six months) for nonpregnant women. As of yet, there is not significant data to show a longer-term benefit.

Probiotics provide beneficial bacteria that colonize the GI tract with optimal amounts and types of bacteria to protect against inflammation and to support immunity and healthy digestive function. In cases where someone is dealing with yeast overgrowth or a histamine intolerance and they want to avoid fermented foods, then a probiotic supplement may sometimes be the best choice.

For those who can tolerate fermented foods, they are an excellent source of natural probiotics that wield powerful microbial properties.

Excellent Probiotic Foods

Yogurt

Kefir

Certain cheeses

Traditional Fermented Foods

Sauerkraut

Pickles

Tempeh

Miso

Kimchi

The Difference between Prebiotics and Probiotics

Prebiotics are nondigestible fibers that encourage the growth of beneficial microbes. Prebiotics, which feed probiotics, help create a colonic environment that is favorable for probiotic vitality. In contrast, probiotics are live colonies of bacteria that promote a more beneficial balance of intestinal flora. Researchers are currently exploring the positive impact of supplemental prebiotics and probiotics on microbial alteration correlating with the onset of an array of chronic conditions that include irritable bowel syndrome (IBS), small intestinal bacterial overgrowth (SIBO), and leaky gut syndrome.

Excellent Prebiotic Foods

Apples
Artichokes
Asparagus
Dandelion greens
Jerusalem artichokes
Jicama root
Onions
Garlic
Leeks
Plantains
Underripe bananas
Cranberries
Pomegranate
Green tea
Seaweed

While the data on probiotics is still under review, one thing is for sure—the gut, bladder, and vaginal (for those with a vagina) microbial ecosystem must be healthy for you to be healthy. Understanding the effect a disruption in the microbiome plays in our overall health is paramount.

What Do We Know?

Our gut bacteria regulate many of our bodily functions, from creating vitamins to regulating our immune system, our brain functions, and of course our metabolism and weight. The microbiome is critical to our long-term health.

Lactobacillus and bifidobacterium are considered the superstars (or maybe we should say "superbugs"), because their abundance is linked to better health outcomes and less risk of chronic diseases like obesity, Alzheimer's disease, type 2 diabetes, and cancer. It demonstrates the importance of being cautious with antibiotic use. For many of my patients, antibiotic use has been a problem in their past: When and if practitioners couldn't properly decipher the ailment, they were given antibiotics that ultimately created resistance patterns and alterations in their microbiome.

Some of the exciting discoveries around the microbiome involve the role of what are called polyphenols, essentially the colorful phytonutrients found in plants. (We discussed much of this in Chapter 12.) The good "bugs" of the microbiome feed on these powerful phytonutrients and in turn provide us with a healthy gut and protection.

For example, there is emerging research that shows a strand of bacteria known as Akkermansia is the next generation of beneficial gut microbes. Akkermansia is thought to feed on the phytonutrients found in cranberries, pomegranate, and green tea. It is thought that when this bacteria is in abundance, it creates a protective layer in the gut that helps prevent symptoms of leaky gut syndrome. It has been linked to positive health outcomes like weight loss, improved insulin resistance, lower inflammation, and more! Many propose that the mechanisms behind interstitial cystitis or bladder pain syndrome are similar to that of leaky gut syndrome, making Akkermansia a microbe I have my eye on. The jury is out, but it sounds like there may be potential for very good things ahead!

MINDFULNESS AND PAIN

Practice makes neuroplasticity.

Everyday stressors have more of an impact on the body than most of us realize. Once stressors are identified, the brain begins to put the body into a state of fight or flight. This stress causes real, physical effects in the body.

Over time, the brain and central nervous system learn to continue to put the body into a painful state, which repeats the pain cycle.

As mindfulness meditation is being introduced into the mainstream to help combat pain, many questions are surfacing about whether it really helps, and about the exact mechanisms by which it might provide some benefit.

The start of the mindfulness movement in the West was first introduced by Jon Kabat-Zinn, who was one of the first to study the association between mindfulness meditation and pain. One of the first studies was done in 1985, and it looked at 90 chronic pain patients who utilized Mindfulness Based Stress Reduction (MBSR). The results of this study were groundbreaking in the realm of chronic pain, showing statistically significant reductions in measures of pain, mood disturbance, and psychological changes, including anxiety and depression. Additionally, pain-related drug utilization was reduced. Since that study, there have been many more with similar findings. I believe it is safe to say that the importance of mindfulness in managing chronic pain is undeniable.

The mechanisms behind how mindfulness reduces pain is really done by attuning the sensation of pain with the subjective judgment we attach to pain as it relates to our perception. Read that again.

Pain is a complex phenomenon, mainly due to it being a multifactorial and subjective experience that consists of sensory, physical, and cognitive elements. Meaning, when we first experience a sensation of pain, we begin to judge it as bad and as something we want to immediately eradicate. We then start to conspire ways to escape the pain, to find any solution we can come up with, all the while continuing to judge our pain as negative. The subjective judgment we add inflates the pain, making the experience of it far more noxious than the sensory experience alone. Think about placing your hand on a stove: It becomes hot and painful. You remove your hand from the triggering event, of course. But what happens to our awareness of the pain? It increases. It becomes entirely more painful. Part of this is physiologic and is due to the firing of the affected sensory and pain neurons, but the other part of this is a cycle of what we feel toward this event, making the feeling of pain even worse.

The goal of mindfulness meditation is to create more awareness of the sensation of pain itself, without judgment or resistance. The presence of pain and our response to it creates a cycle, and this cycle can lead to psychological sequelae like depression and anxiety.

When we become more *aware* of what we are actually experiencing without the overlay of judgments, our perception of pain is changed.

While focusing on the sensory experience of pain could sound counterproductive, it actually provides a pathway to pain relief that is different than the traditional pharmacologic interventions that aim to quell the sensation of pain immediately. Also remember, because pain is multifactorial in nature, using mindfulness as an adjunctive therapy is helpful in any and all senses.

Mensendieck Somatocognitive Therapy

Somatocognitive therapy is a branch of physiotherapy that bridges the mind-body connection. Building on the principles of functional anatomy and motor learning, as well as cognitive psychotherapy, somatocognitive therapy promotes awareness of your own body and an empathic understanding of your own mental state. Studies have shown that this type of therapy has been especially effective in treating chronic pelvic pain. When compared with control groups who received standard gynecological treatment, women who received somatocognitive therapy saw a 25 to 60 percent improvement in their motor function and a 50 percent reduction in pain symptoms. This suggests that Mensendieck somatocognitive therapy may be more effective at relieving pelvic pain than standard treatment alone. Your doctor may recommend you see a therapist who specializes in this type of therapy to help form a well-rounded plan for your symptoms.

Mindfulness Meditation and Possible Mechanisms of Pain Relief

With the advent of modern imaging techniques such as the functional magnetic resonance imaging (MRI), neuroscientists are finding changes in the brain that are quite intriguing and supportive of the benefits of mindfulness meditation.

- The brains of meditators respond differently to pain: Yes. I said it. One study done in 2011 used MRI to show what occurs in the brain during mindfulness meditation in patients with pain. They found that during pain, meditators (although, presumably, they were in a nonmeditative state while being looked at in the MRI machine) had increased activation in the areas of the brain associated with processing the actual sensory experience of pain (including the primary and secondary somatosensory areas, insula, thalamus, and midcingulate cortex). They also found decreased activity in regions involved in emotion, memory, and appraisal (including the medial prefrontal cortex, amygdala, caudate, and hippocampus).
- Activation of a different neural pathway than a placebo: So let's be real. It ain't fake. Another study found mostly consistent results, and they went a step further and accomplished the feat of proving that mindfulness meditation has a different neural pathway response than a placebo, and meditation reduces pain intensity above and beyond a placebo. In this study, relative to other comparison groups, mindfulness meditation was associated with decreased activity in the

brain area called the thalamus. This possibly reflects the inability of sensory information from reaching areas of the brain associated with thinking and evaluation.

While mindfulness meditation is not the be-all and end-all panacea for pain, there is enough evidence to indicate that mindfulness practice does in fact lead to reductions in pain intensity and unpleasantness, even more so than a placebo. The proof is even in the brain circuitry. In short, mindfulness meditation can be a safe and effective addition to medical treatment options.

Repetition Rewires the Brain

Consistency is key. Our brains thrive on consistency. So investing just five minutes of your time each day for awareness, mindfulness, and reminding yourself that you are safe and loved can be an absolute game changer.

There's actually a name for this phenomena. It's called Hebb's rule. Think of it as, "neurons that fire together rewire together."

Our life experience is a reflection of the thoughts and behaviors we are repeating. An adaptive habit is formed by repetition of that habit. Here's a take-home point: Five minutes of mindfulness a day promotes neuroplasticity more than one hour of practice a week! Repetition is key. Make time, even if it's five minutes, to allow your mind and body to connect and rewire in a way that's adaptive and beneficial to you!

Remember: When practicing mindfulness the goal is not to control, suppress, or stop our thoughts—it is to actually witness them. Mindfulness helps us pay attention to our experiences as they arise, without judging or evaluating them in any way. It's like witnessing a ship passing through the night. This is the essence of mindfulness.

Now hear me out for a moment. When we are able to cultivate a state of clarity in which we suspend judgment, we become witnesses of our present-moment experience.

Sure, there's temptation to judge that experience as good or bad, black or white. However, the art of letting go of this desire to judge helps us see things as they are rather than through the filters of patterned and conditioned ways of thinking.

In this way, we are less likely to mechanically play out old habitual ways of thinking and living. Cultivating our attention allows us to stay present to each moment as it unfolds.

My Meditation Practice

I am not the doctor who will bore you with facts without actually practicing what I preach. When I recommend meditation to my patients I often receive a blank stare or raised eyebrows. Sometimes it's followed by excuses, but more often I'm asked questions about if and how I personally practice meditation. So I tell them. And for me, I should say it is a practice that is continually evolving.

The first portion of my meditation practice happens when I first take a seat. It involves checking in with myself and my thoughts and my feelings right at that moment. I acknowledge their existence, understanding that my next step actually involves taking a step back from them.

It's in this space that I start to become more patient with myself and, therefore, others. I try my best to allow thoughts to pass without attaching or identifying with the endless chatter of the ego, and I focus my meditation practice by counting breaths or focusing on a light, like that of a candle. I tend to have to redirect my thoughts, which only strengthens my practice, noting that feelings of stress and anxiety may be present but temporary.

Cultivating my meditation practice has been a lifelong journey for me. It is one that continues to change. But the basics, they stay the same. I end my practice with a mantra—one that my parents taught me when I first began my plunge into meditation:

Lokah samastah sukhino bhavantu ("May all beings everywhere be happy and free, and may the thoughts, words, and actions of my own life contribute in some way to that happiness and to that freedom for all.")

The Body Scan Meditation

So how can we put this theory and research into actionable guidance for our own lives? One of the most effective mindfulness practices with regard to pain reduction is the body scan technique, which provides us with the ability to identify physical discomfort in different parts of the body.

The body scan can allow us to use our bodies to experience present-centered, nonjudgmental awareness. We can learn to be aware of whatever sensation arises in our bodies, particularly the painful ones, and then we can learn to notice the difference between the direct experience of these sensations and the indirect perceptions we add on to that experience. We can learn to notice our bodies.

The body scan allows us to nonjudgmentally identify what we are feeling and where we are feeling it as we narrow our focus on each detailed part of our bodies. Yet, we also begin to train our minds to broaden our focus away from the intricate body parts to a broader and more spacious awareness of the body as it exists as a whole, with different coexisting parts and sensations. A greater understanding of what our bodies endure allows us the opportunity to see what it feels, to accept it, and to cultivate compassion for it, without immediately judging it or trying to escape it.

Let's start meditating!

1. Take a seat.
2. Check in with yourself and your thoughts and feelings at the moment.
3. Acknowledge their existence.
4. Allow thoughts and feelings to pass without attaching yourself to them (think ships passing in the night waters).
5. Count breaths or focus on a light such as a candle.
6. Consistently redirect your thoughts if needed (this will only strengthen your practice, noting that feelings of stress or anxiety may be present but temporary).

Let's start noticing!

1. Close your eyes. You may notice your feet on the floor, notice the sensations of your feet touching the floor. Notice the weight and pressure, vibration, heat.
2. You can notice your legs against the chair, pressure, pulsing, heaviness, lightness.
3. Notice your back against the chair.
4. Bring your attention into your stomach area. If your stomach is tense or tight, let it soften. Take a breath.

5. Notice your hands. Notice if your hands are tense or tight. See if you can allow them to soften.

6. Notice your arms. Feel any sensation in your arms. Let your shoulders be soft.

7. Notice your neck and throat. Let them be soft. Relax. Unclench your jaw.

8. Soften your jaw. Let your face and facial muscles be soft. Do the same with other parts of your body, including your spine and pelvis.

9. Then notice your whole body present. Take one more breath.

10. Be aware of your whole body as best you can. Take a breath. And then when you're ready, you can open your eyes.

Whether I've convinced you or not, I hope you see how important starting or continuing a mindfulness meditation practice can be in your healing journey, whether or not you suffer from pain. And while practice doesn't always make perfect (because really what is perfection anyway?) you can make progress, gain presence, and of course, neuroplasticity!

AFTERWORD: NOW WHAT?

As I said at the beginning of this book, clinical medicine is constantly changing and this book is not meant to represent a comprehensive cohort of clinical care (either on- or off-label) for every chronic pelvic pain patient.

But I do hope that, having read it, you now better understand the currently understood root causes and treatment strategies for pelvic pain and feel empowered to navigate your own care as medicine evolves.

I encourage you to find a health care provider who values keeping both their clinical practices and procedures up to date and their patients informed about the latest available treatment strategies, and who focuses on creating a holistic treatment plan after uncovering the root cause of your pain.

Your pelvic pain has interfered with your life for long enough.

ACKNOWLEDGMENTS

Thank you to all who helped with this book. This book would not have been possible without the support of my husband, who ensured never-ending cups of coffee during the early, early mornings writing at the computer. And to my kids, who are my constant source of inspiration and humor.

I would also like to thank Amanda Olson, DPT PRPC, and Deborah Kiehlmeier, DO, ABPN, who contributed invaluable information essential to various aspects of this book.

To my publishing team at Countryman Press, thank you all.

GLOSSARY

CBT therapy: CBT, or cognitive behavioral therapy, was created by Aaron Beck and is the most well-researched form of psychotherapy. Due to this, a lot of positive evidence exists about this form of therapy. The theory behind CBT is that we experience negative feelings as a result of our perception of events, which does not always align with what factually occurred. Aaron Beck theorized that this negative misinterpretation begins with one's core beliefs, which generally develop during childhood. Core beliefs are deeply held beliefs about the self, others, and the world. These core beliefs may be false and lead to dysfunctional assumptions, which then led to negative automatic thoughts. Subsequently, by challenging your core beliefs when appropriate, you may begin to feel better. CBT is a beneficial type of psychotherapy for many individuals.

DBT therapy: DBT, or dialectic behavior therapy, was created by Marsha Linehan. Marsha Linehan was misdiagnosed as schizophrenic and went through extensive mental health treatment before she self-diagnosed with borderline personality disorder. She created DBT as a modified version of CBT specifically for treating borderline personality disorder. DBT is different from CBT as it is based on acceptance of feelings instead of trying to alter them. With acceptance of feelings, one can then focus on changing their behaviors that are contributing to their distress. Another way DBT differs from other therapies is that it is generally done in a group setting, because it is believed that individuals with borderline personality disorder benefit from working through their personal issues in that context. DBT has good evidence in treating borderline personality disorder. However, it is also a beneficial treatment for those who suffer from chronic suicidality, eating disorders, mood lability, or impulsive behaviors.

Fibromyalgia: Fibromyalgia is a disorder characterized by widespread musculoskeletal pain accompanied by fatigue, sleep, memory, and mood issues. Primary symptoms of fibromyalgia include widespread pain, fatigue, and cognitive difficulties. Researchers believe that fibromyalgia amplifies painful sensations by affecting the way your brain and spinal cord process painful and nonpainful signals. By definition, the pain associated with fibromyalgia must last for at least three months and occur throughout the body, not limited to one side of the body bilaterally. Fibromyalgia often occurs with other comorbid conditions such as irritable bowel syndrome, interstitial cystitis, migraine, depression, and chronic fatigue.

Irritable bowel syndrome: Irritable bowel syndrome (IBS) is a widespread condition involving recurrent abdominal pain and diarrhea or constipation. It's often associated with stress, depression, anxiety, or previous intestinal infection. Signs and symptoms include cramping, abdominal pain, bloating, gas, and diarrhea or constipation, or both.

Lichen sclerosus: Lichen sclerosus is a chronic, inflammatory skin disease that can affect any body part but most often presents in the genitals (penis and vulva). While the cause is unknown, patients can improve with proper individualized treatment.

Lichen planus: Lichen planus is also a chronic, inflammatory, and immune-mediated skin disease that can affect skin, nails, hair, and mucous membranes.

Temporomandibular disorders: Temporomandibular disorders (TMD) are disorders of the jaw muscles, temporomandibular joints, and the nerves associated with chronic facial pain, including TMJ. Any problem that prevents the complex system of muscles, bones, and joints from working together in harmony may result in temporomandibular disorder. TMD is often characterized by chronic pain localized to the jaw that can result in issues with grinding, chewing, and headaches.

Titration: The concept of titrating up medication involves increasing the amount and time with which the medication stays on the vestibule. Often with an individualized approach, we are able to slowly increase this over time as the patient habituates to the medication.

TMS therapy: TMS, or transcranial magnetic stimulation, is an FDA-approved treatment option for depression. TMS occurs through a medical device that applies electrical pulses to the brain using a magnetic coil that is placed over the head. Psychiatrists generally consider referring patients for TMS if they believe they have treatment-resistant depression that has not responded to multiple psychotropic medications. In an initial TMS appointment, the patient's brain structure is mapped, which allows for assessment of areas that should be targets for treatment. After that, patients usually begin an initial round of TMS treatments, which generally involves being treated multiple times a week for several weeks straight. TMS is a noninvasive treatment and studies show it has fewer side effects than most standard depression treatments. However, it is not as efficacious as other options for treatment-resistant depression. These other options include procedures such as ECT (electroconvulsive therapy) and drugs like ketamine.

Vulvar vestibule: The vulvar vestibule extends from inside the labia minora at Hart's line to the remnants of the hymenal ring at the vaginal opening, or introitus, and contains the openings of the greater vestibular glands (Bartholin's glands) and lesser vestibular glands (Skene's glands).

PELVIC ANATOMY

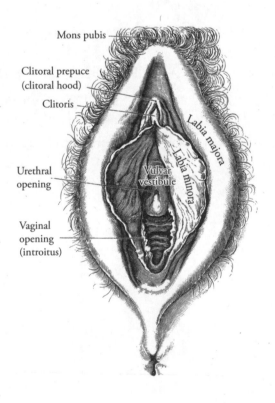

Mons pubis

Clitoral prepuce
(clitoral hood)

Clitoris

Labia majora

Labia minora

Urethral
opening

Vulvar
vestibule

Vaginal
opening
(introitus)

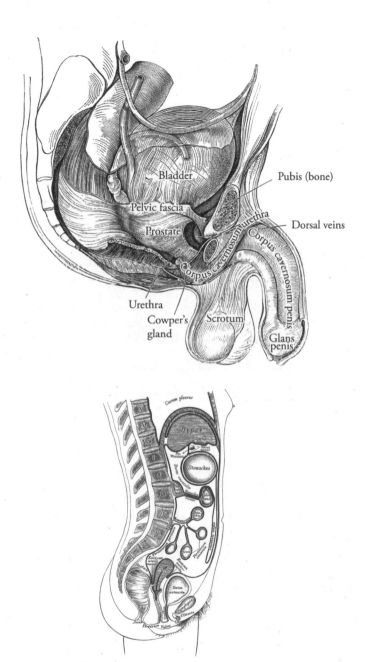

The lower abdomen and pelvic region

RESOURCES

Abbot, J.M., and C. Byrd-Bredbenner. "The State of the American Diet: How Can We Cope?" *Topics in Clinical Nutrition* 22, no. 3 (July 2007): 202–33. DOI: 10.1097/01 .TIN.0000285376.93593.0a.

Abraham, A.D., E.J.Y. Leung, B.A. Wong, et al. "Orally Consumed Cannabinoids Provide Long-Lasting Relief of Allodynia in a Mouse Model of Chronic Neuropathic Pain." *Neuropsychopharmacology* 45, no. 7 (June 2019): 1105–14. DOI: 10.1038/s41386-019-0585-3.

Breidt, F., R.F. McFeeters, I. Perez-Diaz, et al. "Fermented Vegetables." In *Food Microbiology: Fundamentals and Frontiers*, edited by M.P. Doyle and R.L. Buchanan. 4th ed. Washington, DC: ASM Press, 2012.

Committee on Advancing Pain Research, Care, and Education; Board on Health Sciences Policy; Institute of Medicine. "A Call for Cultural Transformation of Attitudes Toward Pain and Its Prevention and Management." *Journal of Pain & Palliative Care Pharmacotherapy* 25, no. 4 (2011): 365–69. DOI: 10.3109/15360288.2011.621516.

Di Mascio, P., S. Kaiser, and H. Sies. "Lycopene as the Most Efficient Biological Carotenoid Singlet Oxygen Quencher." *Archives of Biochemistry and Biophysics* 274, no. 2 (November 1989): 532–38. DOI: 10.1016/0003-9861(89)90467-0.

Esposito, K., F. Nappo, F. Giugliano, et al. "Effect of Dietary Antioxidants on Postprandial Endothelial Dysfunction Induced by a High-Fat Meal in Healthy Subjects." *The American Journal of Clinical Nutrition* 77, no. 1 (January 2003): 139–43. DOI: 10.1093/ajcn/77.1.139.

Friedlander, J.I., B. Shorter, and R.M. Moldwin. "Diet and Its Role in Interstitial Cystitis/Bladder Pain Syndrome (IC/BPS) and Comorbid Conditions." *BJU International* 109, no. 11 (June 2012): 1584–91. DOI: 10.1111/j.1464-410X.2011.10860.x.

Gilbert, B.R. *Medical Acupuncture: A Primer.* New York: Weill-Cornell Medical College, 2002.

Glazer, H.I., and W.J. Ledger. "Clinical Management of Vulvodynia." Review. Gynaecological Practice 2, no. 1–2 (September 2002): 83–90. DOI: 10.1016/S1471-7697(02)00018-7.

Goldstein, A.T., C.F. Pukall, and I. Goldstein, eds. *Female Sexual Pain Disorders: Evaluation and Management.* 2nd ed. Hoboken, NJ: Wiley-Blackwell, 2020.

Hanno, P.M., J.R. Landis, Y. Matthews-Cook, et al. "The Diagnosis of Interstitial Cystitis Revisited: Lessons Learned from the National Institutes of Health Interstitial Cystitis Database Study." *The Journal of Urology* 161, no. 2 (February 1999): 553–57. DOI: 10.1016/s0022-5347(01)61948-7.

Kabat-Zinn, J. *Full Catastrophe Living: Using the Wisdom of Your Body and Mind to Face Stress, Pain, and Illness.* New York: Dell Publishing, 1991.

Moldwin, R.M., ed. *Urological and Gynaecological Chronic Pelvic Pain: Current Therapies.* New York: Springer, 2017.

Morley, S., C. Eccleston, and A. Williams. "Systemic Review and Meta-Analysis of Randomized Controlled Trials of Cognitive Behaviour Therapy and Behaviour Therapy for Chronic Pain in Adults, Excluding Headache." *Pain* 80, no. 1 (March 1999): 1–13. DOI: 10.1016/S0304-3959(98)00255-3.

Nickel, J.C., D. Shoskes, and K. Irvine-Bird. "Clinical Phenotyping of Women with Interstitial Cystitis/Painful Bladder Syndrome: A Key to Classification and Potentially Improved Management." *The Journal of Urology* 182, no. 1 (July 2009): 155–60. DOI: 10.1016/j.juro.2009.02.122.

Peters, K.M. "Interstitial Cystitis—Is It Time to Look Beyond the Bladder?" *The Journal of Urology* 187, no. 2 (February 2012): 381–82. DOI: 10.1016/j.juro.2012.09.020.

Pundir, J., K. Omanwa, E. Kovoor, et al. "Laparoscopic Excision versus Ablation for Endometriosis-Associated Pain: An Updated Systematic Review and Meta-Analysis." *Journal of Minimally Invasive Gynecology* 24 no. 5 (July–August 2017): 747–56. DOI: 10.1016/j.jmig.2017.04.008.

Shorter, B., M. Lesser, R.M. Moldwin, et al. "Effect of Comestibles on Symptoms of Interstitial Cystitis." *The Journal of Urology* 178, no. 1 (July 2007): 145–52. DOI: 10.1016/j.juro.2007.03.020.

Shoskes, D.A., and J.C. Nickel. "Quercetin for Chronic Prostatitis/Chronic Pelvic Pain Syndrome." *Urologic Clinics of North America* 38, no. 3 (August 2011): 279–84. DOI: 10.1016/j.ucl.2011.05.003.

Tall, J.M., and S.N. Raja. "Dietary Constituents as Novel Therapies for Pain." *The Clinical Journal of Pain* 20, no. 1 (January–February 2004): 19–26. DOI: 10.1097/00002508-200401000-00005.

Thilakarathna, S.H., and H.P. Vasantha Rupasinghe. "Flavonoid Bioavailability and Attempts for Bioavailability Enhancement." *Nutrients* 5, no. 9 (September 2013): 3367–87. DOI: 10.3390/nu5093367.

Worthington, V. "Nutritional Quality of Organic versus Conventional Fruits, Vegetables, and Grains." *The Journal of Alternative and Complementary Medicine* 7, no. 2 (April 2001): 161–73. DOI: 10.1089/107555301750164244.

Wright, J., H. Lotfallah, K. Jones, et al. "A Randomized Trial of Excision versus Ablation for Mild Endometriosis," *Fertility and Sterility* 83, no. 6 (June 2005): 1830–36. DOI: 10.1016/j.fertnstert.2004.11.066.

Zhang, R., L. Lao, K. Ren, et al. "Mechanisms of Acupuncture-Electroacupuncture on Persistent Pain." *Anesthesiology* 120, no. 2 (February 2014): 482–503. DOI: 10.1097/ALN.0000000000000101.

INDEX

Bladder, 3, 35
cancer of, 35
cannabidiol for, 175
disorders of, 131
glycosaminoglycan layer of,
6, 33, 100, 116
irritants in, 134–135
persistent urgency in, 61
stones in, 35
Bladder instillations, 99–103
in treating interstitial cystitis, 36
Bladder pain, 31, 65
hormones and, 68
Bladder pain syndrome, 5, 26,
31, 32, 72, 131. *See also*
Interstitial cystitis
cystoscopy in diagnosing,
35–36
living with, 37
treating, 100, 101
Blocking reuptake, 88
Body scan, breathing with,
166–168
Body scan meditation,
190–191
Botox, 103, 105–107, 155
in treating pelvic floor
dysfunction, 51, 53
in treating pudendal neuralgia, 59
Botulinum toxin A, adverse
effects of, 106
Bowel, 3
disorders in, 132
Bowel-bladder connection, 112
Bowel-bladder convergence,
126
Bowel movements, 5
Brain, exercise in helping
function, 140–141
Brain-derived neurotrophic
factor (BDNF), 140
Breathing
with body scan or reduced
tension, 166–168
deep, for pelvic pain,
165–168
diaphragmatic, 171
yoga and, 146–147
Breath work, 168–172
for life, 172
utilizing, 168–169
Bulbospongiosus muscle, 45
Bupivacaine, 101, 105

Burning, 23
B vitamins, 115

Caffeine, in preventing endometriosis, 78–79
Cancer, 77
of the bladder, 35
endometriosis-associated
adenocarcinoma and, 77
Candidiasis, vulvovaginal, 180,
181
Cannabidiol (CBD), 172–180
intoxicating or mental status
altering effect of, 177
lubricants, 177, 178, 179
questions and answers
regarding, 175–177
sex and, 177–178
types of, 176
Capsaicin, 99
Carcinogens, 111
Carotenoid, 111
Case studies
Barbara, 52–53
Caitlynn, 80–81
Josh, 151–152
Cat and cow flow, 136
Cave squat, 136
CBT (cognitive behavioral
therapy) therapy, 11, 196
Cell transformations, 75
Central sensitization, 64
Cesarean section, 132
Child's pose, 135–136, **148**
Chronic fatigue, 197
Chronic overlapping pain
conditions, 40
Chronic pain, 3, **12**, 40, 50
Chronic pain syndrome, 126
Chronic prostatitis/chronic
pelvic pain, 151
Clinical medicine, as con-
stantly changing, ix
Clitoris, 55, 67, **200**
Coating agents, 101
Coccydynia, 132, 159
Coccygeus muscle, 45
Cognitive behavior therapy
(CBT), 11, 196
Colposcope, 44
Comorbid chronic pain condi-
tions, 40, 72
Confirmation bias, 17–19
Constipation, 132

Constipation supplements,
124–125
Cortisol, 140
Cowper's glands, 66, **201**
Creams, 93
Cromolyn, 96
Cross talk, 63–64
Cupping, 153
Cyclobenzaprine, 90
Cystitis. *See* Interstitial cystitis
Cystoscopy in diagnosing inter-
stitial cystitis/bladder
pain syndrome, 35–36
Cysts
Bartholin's, 97
ovarian, 76
sebaceous, 97

D-mannose, 122
Decompression surgery, in
treating pudendal neu-
ralgia, 60
Deep breathing, for pelvic
pain, 165–168
Depression, 9, 11, 14
Detoxification, 111
Dialectic behavior therapy
(DBT), 11, 196–197
Diaphragm, 147
Diaphragmatic breathing, 171
Diazepam, 90
Diet. *See also* Food; Nutrition
changes in, in preventing
endometriosis, 79
elimination, 116–119
fads and, 118–119
increasing whole grains in,
115–116
link between pelvic pain
and, 112–116
role of, in pelvic pain, 110
well-being and, 109
Diet therapy, 154
Digestive system, 3
Dilators, 158–165
Dimethyl sulfoxide (DMSO), 102
Dioxins, 75
Distress, 11
Drowsiness, 139
Dry needling, 104, 105
Due diligence, 21
Dysmenorrhea, 62
Dyspareunia, 132
Dyssynergia, 5, 49

INDEX

Interstitial cystitis, 31, 40, 72, 131, 132, 175
age and, 34
causes of, 32–34
chronic inflammation in, 110
cystoscopy in diagnosing, 35–36
diagnosing, 34–35
gender and, 34
need for cystoscopy in diagnosing, 35–36
pelvic floor physical therapy in treating, 36
referred pain in, 62
skin and hair color and, 34
symptoms of, 5–6, 32, 122
treating, 36–37, 100
Intra-abdominal pressure (IAP), 147
Involuntary guarding, 50
Irritable bowel syndrome (IBS), 26, 33, 34, 40, 72, 110, 132, 182, 197–198
chronic inflammation in, 110, 182
fibromyalgia and, 197–198
in men, 26, 34
in women, 132
Isocyanates, 111

Journaling, 141–142

Kabat-Zinn, Jon, 184
Kaempferol, 111
Kegel exercises, 134
Ketamine, 199

Labia, 55, **200**
labia majora, 39, 97, **200**
labia minora, 39, 67, 69, 97, **200**
Lactobacillus, 69, 183
Lactobacillus reuteri, 126
Lactobacillus rhamnosus, 126
Laparoscopy, 132
Leaky gut, 6
Leaky gut syndrome, 126, 182
symptoms of, 184
Legs up the wall, 148
Legumes, 115
Lesions, Hunner's, 36
Lesser vestibular glands, 199
Lethargy, 139

Levator ani syndrome, 44, 132
Lichen planus, 96, 132, 198
Lichen sclerosis, 44, 96, 132, 198
Lichen simplex chronicus, 44
Lidocaine, 101, 105
Lifestyle changes and modifi-cations, 137–144
exercise in, 139–141
journaling in, 141–142
sleep in, 138–139
standing desks in, 143
stress management in, 142–143
in treating interstitial cystitis, 36
in treating pudendal neural-gia, 59
vulvar hygiene in, 143–144
Linehan, Marsha, 196–197
Littré, gland of, 66
Lumbar plexus, 107
Lutein, 112
Lycopene, 111
Lymphatic system transport, 76
Lymphedema, 132

Magnesium, 115, 125
Magnetic resonance imaging (MRI), 187
Massage, 154
Mast cell degranulation, treat-ing, 100
Mast cell inhibitors, 96
Mayer-Rokitansky-Küster (MRKH) syndrome, 163
Medications. *See also specific*
oral, 45, 59, 87–91
antidepressants as, 86, 87–89
antihistamines as, 91
gabapentin as, 89–90
muscle relaxers as, 90–91
in treating pudendal neural-gia, 59
tropical, 45, 91–103
amitriptyline-based prepa-rations as, 95–96
capsaicin as, 99
cromolyn as, 96
gabapentin as, 94–95
hormones as, 93–94
lidocaine as, 98

Meditation
body scan, 190–191
mindfulness, 187–188
Melatonin, 139
Menopause, 68–70
Mensendieck somatocognitive therapy, 186
Menstruation, retrograde, 75
Mental health effects, 77
Methocarbamol, 90
Microbiome, 112, 142
vaginal, 69
Microbiota-gut-brain axis, 142
Migraine, 105, 197
Mindfulness, 184–192
Mindfulness Based Stress Reduction (MBSR), 184–185
Mindfulness meditation, 187–188
Mons pubis, **200**
Muscle memory, 129
Muscle relaxants for pelvic floor dysfunction, 21, 53
Muscle relaxers, 90–91
Myofascial trigger points, 104

Needling, 105, 155
dry, 104, 105
Nerve blocks, 103, 107–108, 155
Nerves, 54–64, 107
ganglion impar, 107
genitofemoral, 107
iliohypogastric, 107
ilioinguinal, 107
lumbar plexus, 107
pudendal, 54–55, 107, 171
superior hypogastric plexus, 107
trigeminal, 170, 171
vagus, 169–171
Nerve stimulation
in treating interstitial cystitis, 36
in treating pudendal neural-gia, 60
Neural sensitization, 100
Neurogenic inflammation, treating, 100
Neurogenic upregulation, 33
Neuromuscular disorders, 26
Neuropathic pain, treating, 89

207